Medical Cost Crisis

Other books by Don W. Larson

Land of the Giants
The Onan Story

Medical Cost Crisis

A Common-Sense Solution

Don W. Larson

Bond Publishing

Published by:
Bond Publishing Co.
537 East Vine Street
Owatonna, Minnesota 55060
1-800-374-6888

ISBN 0-9635576-0-2

Printed in the United States of America
10 9 8 7 6 5 4 3 2 1

This book is dedicated to my dear wife and very best friend, Geil, and our four wonderful children, Mark, Brad, Jil, and Steve, and their families.

To contact the publisher:
Bond Publishing Co.
537 East Vine Street
Owatonna, MN 55060

TOLL FREE PHONE NUMBER:
1-800-374-6888

To contact the author directly:
(507) 455-3220

Foreward

After more than five years of research into this country's health-care problems, reading nearly a hundred books and thousands of newspaper and magazine articles on the subect, I am amazed only about one thing:

Why has no one else come up with a solution similar to the one outlined in this book?

My "Common-Sense Solution" to our medical care crisis is not a radical proposal. It is simple, workable, and will cost far less than our current system with no decline in quality of health care. It also will make medical services available to everyone in the nation at affordable expense.

I feel certain someone in this huge country has, in the past, suggested a similar solution, and I have just missed it, but it obviously isn't a widely touted proposal.

Concerned that my solution must contain some horrendous flaw, I have presented the concept to dozens of very knowledgeable Americans, including U.S. senators, physicians, hospital administrators, business leaders and ordinary consumers. Not one raised serious objections to the proposal.

Perhaps the "Common-Sense Solution" is too simple to be accepted by the brilliant people who have come up with more than a hundred complex proposals to reform our health-care system.

Unfortunately, all these other "solutions" have several things in common: They will result in much higher costs, they will result in rationing of medical care, and they will make our current system even worse.

There's little question that some type of reform is inevitable, but the only way my solution will gain consideration is by action from you and other readers of this book.

If my "Common-Sense Solution" appeals to you as workable and the proper way to fix a broken system, it will be necessary for you to carry the message to others.

Otherwise, be prepared to have a continuation of a very serious medical cost crisis.

Contents

Contents

Understanding the Problem

1

You have just finished a grueling 10-hour day at your office, and you are tired, hungry and a bit crabby. Your wife and children are visiting relatives out of town, so you decide to treat yourself to a big, delicious steak at a restaurant.

Although you haven't been there before, you know of a nearby restaurant that features a huge, juicy steak on Thursday nights. When you arrive, you see the "special" scrawled on a blackboard just inside the front door. The sign reads: "12-ounce T-bone steak, french fries, vegetable, beverage and dessert of your choice."

No price is listed, but you don't even bother to ask about it. You just order the "special" and wait for your dinner.

Shortly after you start eating, you notice three other people at nearby tables also enjoying the restaurant's "special" of the day. One is a man dressed in a business suit and tie, another is a gray-haired woman who reminds you of your grandmother, and the other is a middle-aged man who looks as if he bought his ill-fitting, rumpled clothes from a second-hand store.

You enjoy your meal, and when you finish you go to the front of the restaurant where the manager is standing behind a counter next to a cash register.

The other three patrons who had the same steak "special" as yours are already in line. You stand at the end of the line, and you hear the restaurant manager tell the man in the rumpled clothes that his bill is $4.10. You think to yourself, "Wow, what a bargain!" Then you hear the manager charge the older woman $6.50, and you wonder what's going on. When the man in the business suit is charged $11.75, you quickly glance at your bill and angrily notice it reads $35.

You confront the manager: "What kind of a scam are you pulling here. We all had the same meal, but we all have to pay different amounts."

The manager sheepishly explains to you that he has no control over the different prices being charged. He says, "The first man is poor and is on welfare, and the state government won't allow me to charge him more than $4.10. The woman is over 65 years old, and she belongs to the federal program called Medicafe, which mandates what I can charge her. The other guy is in a business group that has negotiated lower rates. If I charge him more than these rates, I lose all of the group's business."

The manager goes on: "You, on the other hand, don't fit into any of these categories, so I have to charge you $35 to make up for the losses I'm forced to take on these other people. Sorry about that."

Don't laugh. You most likely think this outrageous pricing system is entirely too weird to ever happen, and, if it did, it would quickly destroy the country's dining-out industry.

But this is exactly how health care is priced throughout the United States, and if this several-tier pricing mechanism is allowed to continue, you can expect some tragic consequences in the quality of treatment provided by irate doctors and hospitals.

As an example, let's look at how the Stanford University Medical Center in California is required to price coronary bypass surgery. This is a very expensive and complicated procedure performed on patients with clogged arteries leading to the heart. Another vessel from the patient, most often from the leg, is used to circumvent the plugged arteries near the heart.

It was reported recently in the *Wall Street Journal* that it costs the Stanford center from $35,000 to $41,000 for its surgeons to perform a coronary bypass, but Medicare (the federal insurance program for people 65 and older) allows a charge of only $27,000 for the operation. And Medicaid, the joint federal-state program to assist poor people, will permit a paltry charge of only $11,000.

If you have private insurance or are uninsured, the Stanford center has to charge you $81,000 for the operation, according to the *Journal* article.

In an attempt to fight this ridiculous pricing system, which is rampant throughout the country, many large corporations and insurance companies are now shopping around for medical prices that are closer to those being paid by government programs. This merely makes the expense for the rest of us even higher.

Although cost shifting is only one of many problems in the current U.S. medical-care crisis, it is an excellent example of how efforts to reform the system have only made it worse.

Attempts by the government, large companies and even groups of smaller businesses to force price controls on medical-care providers are simply not working. They not only shift costs to people without clout, but they encourage shenanigans by doctors and hospitals that are responsible for some of today's soaring costs.

And soaring they are!

Total costs for all types of health care in the U.S. for 1993 are expected to exceed an unbelievable 900 billion dollars (see table on Page 5), almost

TOTAL ANNUAL COST OF HEALTH CARE

(From U.S. Health Care Financing Administration)

YEAR	BILLIONS	PERCENT OF GNP	ANNUAL INCREASE	INFLA-TION
1993*	$906.3	13.8%	10.9%	3.7%
1992	817.2	13.2	10.7	3.5
1991	737.9	12.4	10.8	3.1
1990	666.2	12.2	10.5	6.1
1989	602.8	11.8	10.4	4.5
1988	546.0	11.2	10.5	4.4
1987	494.1	11.0	8.6	4.4
1986	454.8	10.6	7.6	1.1
1985	422.6	10.3	9.2	3.8
1984	387.0	10.7	9.0	3.9
1983	355.0	10.3	10.9	3.8
1982	320.0	10.1	10.0	3.8
1981	291.0	9.5	16.4	8.9
1980	250.1	9.1	13.2	12.5
1979	221.0	8.6	10.5	13.3
1978	200.0	8.4	11.1	9.0
1977	180.0	8.4	20.0	6.7
1976	150.0	8.5	7.1	4.9
1975	140.0	8.4	27.3	6.9
1974	110.0	8.0	10.0	12.3
1973	100.0	7.4	6.4	8.7
1972	94.0	7.7	16.1	3.4
1971	81.0	7.3	8.9	3.3
1970	74.4	7.2	9.4	5.6
1965	41.0	5.9		
1960	27.1	5.3		
1950	13.5	4.7		
1940	4.0	4.0		
1930	3.5	3.5		

*projected

double what we spent in 1986. And projections for the year 2000 show that total costs will soar to about 1.5 trillion dollars, which is more than the federal government is currently spending for all services—defense, Social Security, welfare, and the hundreds of other programs funded by taxpayers.

The country's health-care costs today are consuming nearly 14 percent of the Gross National Product (GNP), which is the nation's total economic output. Without a drastic overhaul of the system, the cost of medical services will consume more than one-quarter of GNP by the year 2030, according to several studies.

Although today's medical costs are paid mostly by private insurance companies and government programs, Americans are fooling themselves if they don't realize that ultimately the entire expense comes out of their pockets.

While individuals currently pay only a small percentage of total charges directly to health-care providers through out-of-pocket disbursements, they pay all of the remainder through taxes, insurance premiums, lower wages, and higher prices for goods and services.

So, if you divide the total health-care costs for 1993 by the number of people living in the United States, you discover that it is costing every man, woman and child in America the staggering sum of $3,625 annually. For a family of four that's $14,500.

These are averages, of course, and can be misleading. A few American families incur annual medical services that cost far more than the average, while most families receive few, if any, actual services in a given year. (This is the key to solving the problem of soaring costs, as you will learn in later chapters.) The significant fact is that 10 percent of the U.S. population—those with serious illnesses or expensive chronic conditions—account for more than half of all health-care costs.

To better understand why medical costs in the U.S. have jumped completely out of control, it's necessary to take a close look at some recent history. The spiraling trend started back in 1965, the year the federal government stuck its ugly foot in the door by implementing the Medicare and Medicaid programs.

Designed to help older citizens, the poor and disabled pay for their medical bills, both programs went into effect in 1966, and ever since then total health-care costs have leaped by two to three times the rate of inflation in nearly every year.

Back in 1965, the federal government spent only 1.8 percent of its total budget on health care, while today it is more than 15 percent and rising constantly. In 1965, when total health-care costs were $41 billion, the amount represented only 5.9 percent of the country's Gross National Product. In 1940, a quarter of a century earlier, total costs were 4 percent of GNP, not much different from 25 years later.

Since 1965, however, it has been a vastly different scenario. Costs, measured as a percent of GNP, more than doubled in the next 25 years, and they soon will triple the 1965 percentage.

Some people contend that roaring inflation is a major cause of rising health-care costs. Wrong! If total medical expenses had increased at the rate of inflation between 1965 and 1993, they would have climbed from $40 billion to $183.9 billion. Instead, the 1993 costs will be $906.3 billion. That means $722.4 billion of the increase is due to reasons other than inflation.

What has gone wrong? Has the quality of medical care improved so dramatically that it costs much more to treat patients? Have physicians and other professionals increased their compensation beyond comprehension? Are hospitals and other institutions reaping obscene profits?

The answers are no, no, no.

The decision by government to play a major role in health care has been an important factor in rising costs, but there are many other reasons for the industry to act like a speeding, runaway freight train.

The main culprits in this national crisis are what medical-care providers refer to contemptuously as "third-party players." These include federal and state government bureaucrats, health insurance companies, utilization reviewers, cost-containment commissions, actuaries, claims processors, employee benefit plan administrators, attorneys and others whose pretentious role is to regulate the proper amount of medical care and its cost.

In the 200 years prior to 1965, medical care in America was an uncomplicated system with decisions arrived at between the doctor and patient. Costs during this period remained relatively constant. Since 1965, the role of third-party players has grown immensely, and, not coincidentally, the costs of health care have soared beyond belief.

Before 1965, the medical industry was a market-driven system with consumers greatly influencing the cost of services. Patients paid nearly all the costs to doctors and hospitals, and they made decisions based not only on the need for their medical care but also on the cost.

According to the U.S. Congressional Research Service, back in the early 1960s private-sector payments for health care constituted nearly 76 percent of all expenditures, most of which consisted of out-of-pocket spending by consumers.

Today, however, consumers are playing a minor role in the payment system. According to the U.S. Health Care Financing Administration, consumers are paying only 21.2 percent of total costs through out-of-pocket payments for drugs, insurance deductibles, co-payments and other direct expenditures to health-care providers.

Because insurance firms and government programs are paying for the bulk of health care, consumers today have the ill-conceived notion that medical services are predominantly "free."

This attitude has led to many of the costly abuses in today's delivery of health services. Consumers have lost their propensity to control costs, and health-care providers have been forced to play distasteful games with the third-party players over how much to charge for their goods and services.

Of all the factors driving up expenses, the illogical impression that no one is hurt by the medical charges is the most harmful.

The most common expression in doctors' offices, hospitals and other medical facilities is, "Don't worry about it. Your insurance will cover it." This naturally leads to a great amount of unnecessary health care at all facilities throughout the country.

Estimates of the amount of unnecessary health care range from 30 percent to more than 50 percent. Is there any wonder that medical costs are out of control?

Dr. C. Everett Koop, the former U.S. surgeon general, remarked at a health forum in Minneapolis recently, "I truly believe that 30 percent of current diagnostic and treatment procedures are medically unnecessary." Other experts think the amount of unnecessary medical services is even higher than 30 percent.

Milliman & Robertson, Inc., a Seattle-based health-care consulting firm, has estimated that 53 percent of current health-care costs are "medically unnecessary." The company said a recent study has found that 24 percent of U.S. hospital admissions were found to be unwarranted.

Much of this unneeded treatment is due to the unconcerned attitude of consumers, who feel that as long as their insurance companies will pay the bill, there is no need to be wary.

There also is a large number of unnecessary services being performed in the guise of "defensive medicine," which is nothing more than a scandalous method to help protect health-care providers from malpractice lawsuits.

Doctors and hospital officials are well aware of the desperate need to protect themselves from ambitious attorneys who sue at the drop of a surgeon's glove. Each year there are more than 330,000 malpractice suits filed against health-care providers.

Costly and unnecessary "defensive medicine" is used to minimize the impact of possible lawsuits.

A huge number of medical tests and procedures ordered every day by physicians are not for the benefit of the patient but to satisfy the demands of attorneys who defend health-care providers in malpractice litigation.

Dr. Harrison L. Rogers, Jr., former president of the American Medical Society, has defined "defensive medicine" with this statement: "Those tests, procedures and consultants that I order not based on the need of my patient, but on the need to create a paper trail behind me, so that if I'm called to court to discuss a patient of my own or someone else's, I can be certain that I have ordered every possible test that I can be asked about in court."

Ironically, much of the unneeded medical care is caused by peculiar rules and regulations imposed by government officials and other third-party players in their futile attempts to "control" costs.

Here are some actual examples of how these absurd rules can backfire:

A 13-year-old boy falls off his skateboard and hits his head on the concrete sidewalk. He seems dazed and confused, so his grandfather, who was caring for the boy, drives him to a hospital emergency unit. A physician examines the lad and says he can't detect anything, but a CAT (computerized axial tomography) scan would reveal if there was anything seriously wrong.

The grandfather says to go ahead, but the doctor says the rules won't allow him to do so. The doctor says a CAT scan isn't authorized unless the patient was involved in a motorcycle accident or is delivered to the hospital in an ambulance.

The infuriated grandfather tells the doctor to forget it. Having already paid several thousand dollars in insurance premiums in recent months, he wasn't about to pay another $500 out of his pocket for the test. He takes the boy home.

Several hours later, the youngster still has not recovered, so the grandfather calls an ambulance and the boy is given the CAT scan at the hospital. The test shows no permanent damage, and the next morning the boy is fully recovered.

The result is that the episode cost $300 (for the ambulance ride) more than was necessary.

A second example: an elderly woman goes to her physician's office with a difficult-to-control arrhythmia (her heart rate is too fast). The doctor determines he can treat her as an outpatient with a medication to slow the heart rate, but he knows she will require careful medical monitoring several times a week until it's under control.

Medicare rules, however, will not pay for more than one visit a week at the doctor's office, and she needs several. The solution? The doctor puts her in a hospital, where he can check her progress frequently. She doesn't want to go to the hospital and the doctor doesn't feel it's necessary, but the rules require it.

Several thousand dollars are spent unnecessarily on the woman's treatment because of the government's attempt to "control" costs.

Another example of the bungling by third-party players is best told in the words of an actual health-care provider who puts up with such non-sense on a daily basis.

Eileen Weber is a staff nurse at a hospital emergency department in Minneapolis. She wrote the following poignant account, which appeared in the Minneapolis *Star Tribune* on Jan. 12, 1992:

"The paramedic walked her in from the ambulance to the Emergency Department triage area, motioning her to sit down in the screened-off area to the side of the nurse's deck.

"Walking over to me, he rather disgustedly gave me his ambulance run sheet to sign, thereby acknowledging my acceptance of this patient.

" 'Whatcha got?' I asked.

" 'She needs to have her prescription filled,' he replied, anticipating my response to this apparently flagrant abuse of our advanced life support emergency medical system.

"I rolled my eyes in disbelief. 'You're kidding! She called 911 to get her prescription filled here in the middle of the night?'

"I'm usually fairly patient with supposed abusers of the system, figuring there must be extenuating circumstances for people to use the emergency room in ways I don't always easily understand, but this was the most outrageous thing I'd heard in a long time. I figured I might have to explain appropriate use of the 911 system to her, as I've done with other patients.

"Instead, she enlightened me. As I sat down with this tired, feverish, middle-aged woman to do a quick physical assessment, I also elicited her version of what brought her to the hospital.

"As she answered my questions, I felt my anger growing. I became furious at an obstructive health-care insurance system which not only abused this woman, but put her in a position to be further maligned for the supposed 'abuse' this same system drove her to.

"Turns out she had been in a different emergency department the evening before and was diagnosed with a painful kidney infection. Not all people with kidney infections have to be hospitalized, though left untreated they can be lethal, and the emergency room doctor had appropriately discharged her with a prescription for an effective antibiotic. No problem, so far, as her medical assistance was channeled through an HMO (health maintenance organization) that agreed to pay for emergency room visits at the hospital she visited. Dandy idea, this channeling medical assistance (welfare) funds through eager HMOs. Damned efficient.

"Until it came time to get the prescription filled. It is standard practice for folks to be able to get the medicine their doctor prescribes through an in-house pharmacy servicing the emergency department, especially during off hours. Therefore, she had been instructed to go to the hospital pharmacy upon discharge.

"However, once there she couldn't get her medicine unless she paid cash (usually a scarce commodity for welfare patients), because the pharmacy wouldn't get reimbursed by the same HMO which reimburses the emergency room visit. If this befuddles you in your healthy altertness, imagine the frustration this tired, sick woman felt.

"With no other obvious recourse, she went home, where she proceeded to get more feverish and have more pain. As anyone who has suffered pain knows, everything gets worse late at night. In pain, unable to sleep, with no money for medicine, let alone a cab, and with no one to drive her to our hospital, she called for an ambulance. By the time I saw her, she needed to be seen all over again by one of our doctors, not only because our pharmacy can't honor prescriptions from outside doctors, but because she was much more ill. I even called the other hospital's pharmacy to verify this woman's story and to encourage the pharmacist there that he needed to let his supervisor know of this absurdity.

"In order to get the necessary medicine for what is a very easily treated condition, this impoverished woman was forced to visit two expensive emergency departments (complete with waiting times), use an expensive ambulance service (the only kind that responds to 911), generate two separate physician charges, have two sets of blood and urine tests, and get two prescriptions (only one of which was filled).

"What I had before me was another innocent victim of what is probably the most stupid, most wastefully expensive, most classist health-care nonsystem in the industrialized world.

"We who provide care in the emergency setting see this obstructionist idiocy daily. Scratch an emergency nurse or physician with an HMO or a PPO and you will draw boiling blood. Time that should be spent caring for people is spent on the phone pleading with nonmedical secretarial staff (if you're lucky enough to get a non-machine) for permission to get preauthorization. Many folks we see can't read, or English is foreign, or they haven't had the time to wade through all the rules and regulations involved with this 'freedom of choice.'

"Do you, this very instant, know all the deductibles, co-pays, coverage limitations, preferred providers, preauthorization requirements, ambulance coverage, network hospitals, prescription coverage, ad nauseam, of your health 'care' policy?"

Eileen Weber isn't unusual in her feelings about today's overly complicated (and costly) medical-care system, and the examples cited aren't isolated ones. Wasteful and unnecessary treatment is eating up about one-third of total health-care costs, with no relief in sight.

These third-party players also are costing Americans enormous sums in horrendous administrative paperwork in connection with health care.

No one has a good handle on the exact amount wasted as a result of the ever-growing record-keeping that is demanded by insurance companies, government regulators and other third-party players.

There's no question, however, that total costs for all phases of medical bookkeeping, much of which is totally superfluous, is a staggering amount, probably in the neighborhood of $300 billion a year.

Evidence of the tremendous growth of medical record-keeping since 1965 can be found in the amazing increase of people employed in the health-care industry, far exceeding the need due to the population growth or the increase of people requiring treatment.

According to the U.S. Bureau of Census, there were fewer than 4 million workers in the health-care industry in 1965, while today that number has exceeded 10 million. And those 10 million workers do not include pharmacists, school nurses, nurses in private homes, employees of drug companies, medical product companies, health insurance firms, government bureaucrats or other third-party players devoting fulltime to regulating health care.

It has been estimated that one of every 10 Americans is now employed in the health-care industry, and it has become one of the fastest growing fields in the country. One government official has estimated that between 1993 and the year 2000, one of every six new jobs in the U.S. will be in medical care. Most of the jobs are devoted partly or entirely to keeping up with the mushrooming growth of paperwork.

Even the recession of the early 1990s failed to slow the employment growth. The U.S. Bureau of Labor Statistics reported that between June 1990 and January 1992 there was a net increase of 592,000 jobs in the health-care field while there was a net loss of 2.2 million jobs in all industries.

And while the salaries for most jobs in America are showing the smallest gains in 20 years, the wage increases for health-care workers are rising at twice the rate of inflation. A recent study by the Bureau of National Affairs shows that during 1991 the median wage hike in the manufacturing industry was only 3.4 percent, while health-care workers received increases of 6.9 percent.

Unfortunately, there is no evidence the mountain of paperwork required by third-party players has improved the quality of medical care. In fact, it is not only lowering the quality but is a major factor in the soaring costs.

Dr. Sidney Marchasin, vice president of the board of directors at Sequoia Hospital in Redwood City, Calif., summed up the problem succinctly.

He wrote in a guest editorial in the *Wall Street Journal*: "The groans you hear coming from your local hospital are not all emanating from patients. They're the protests of nurses, hospital personnel and physicians who are forced to live with a hodgepodge of expensive, contradictory and confusing bureaucratic regulations. The federal government must be held responsible for many of the basic costs that now confound the health-care industry. Legislators, official commissions and bureaucrats in Washington document deficiencies in our health-care system, point out the need for corrective action, and then invoke all sorts of rules, regulations and paperwork."

Dr. Marchasin has an interesting story to tell about the consequences of mandated, but unnecessary, paperwork at his hospital.

He points out that his hospital today is serving roughly the same number of inpatients as it did in 1966, the year Medicaid and Medicare programs began. He says the hospital currently treats an average of 250 inpatients a day, the same as in 1966.

In 1966, however, the hospital had a total of 448 employees, while today that number has almost doubled, primarily because of the need for all the additional paperwork required.

Dr. Marchasin says the Federal Peer Review Act mandates that all hospital work paid for by the government be reviewed by an independent agency under contract to the Health Care Finance Administration. In addition, to get Medicare payments the hospital must undergo another audit, this one by the Joint Commission on Accreditation of Health Care Organizations. Health insurance companies also require an ever-growing list of authorization forms, patient billings and reviews.

Many of the new employees added by Sequoia Hospital devote all their time to record keeping.

The hospital's business and accounting office has grown from 26 employees to 70. The medical records office now has 41 workers compared with only 17 back in 1966. There are nine workers in the data processing office, 10 in the utilization review office, nine in the social services office, five in the quality assurance office, and four in the medical staff office. None of these departments existed in 1966.

And because nurses at Sequoia now must spend much of their time filling out forms instead of treating patients, the number of nurses on the hospital staff has grown from 374 in 1966 to 533. Nationwide, it has been estimated that nurses devote 50 percent of their duty time performing paperwork.

Dr. Marchasin says, "The price tag for dealing with the various regulatory bodies and government-mandated paperwork at my institution is approximately $7.8 million annually."

Sequoia is an about-average-sized hospital. There are approximately 6,000 hospitals in the U.S., and if each had a similar price tag for administrative paperwork, we are talking about nearly $50 billion a year—just at hospitals.

Physicians and their office workers also face a tremendous bookkeeping task these days, more horrendous even than hospitals. A recent survey showed that each patient's visit to a doctor's office generated from seven to 10 pages of paper, resulting in costs for paper shuffling that were equal to the cost of the doctor's actual medical services.

While employment has nearly doubled at U.S. hospitals during the last two decades, the number of employees at physicians' offices in the nation has just about tripled, while the medical clinics have seen their staffs grow by four times the number employed there in 1970 (see table on Page 24).

While the soaring costs of new rules, regulations and the mountains of paperwork required today of health-care providers are blamed mostly on the federal government and health insurance companies, state governments are equally guilty.

Under various mandated health insurance benefit laws, state governments require insurance companies to constantly expand into areas not traditionally covered by health insurance. In 1970 there were only 48 such state government laws in the U.S. Today there are more than 1,000.

John C. Goodman, president of the National Center for Policy Analysis in Dallas, Texas, says: "Mandated health insurance benefits cover ailments ranging from AIDS to alcoholism and drug abuse, and services ranging from acupuncture to in-vitro fertilization. They cover heart transplants in Georgia, liver transplants in Illinois, hairpieces in Minnesota, marriage counseling in California, pastoral counseling in Vermont and sperm-bank deposits in Massachusetts."

To escape these outrageous state government mandates, many large corporations have elected to self-insure their employees, but this simply makes health care even more costly for taxpayers and those who buy coverage from health insurance companies.

Health-Care Industry Workers*

	1993	1970
Hospitals	4,980,000	2,690,000
Nursing Homes	1,621,000	590,000
Medical Clinics	1,425,000	330,000
Physicians' Offices	1,339,000	477,000
Dentists' Offices	595,000	222,000
Chiropractors' Offices	112,000	19,000
TOTALS:	**10,072,000**	**4,328,000**

*Based on data from U.S. Bureau of Census and U.S. Bureau of Labor Statistics. Not included are pharmacists, school nurses, nurses in private homes, employees of drug companies, medical products companies, health insurance firms, government health workers, private health regulators, or employees of corporations handling health insurance programs.

Solving the Problem

2

Before any complicated problem can be solved, one must fully understand exactly what essential elements are involved and then make certain that any proposed solution improves those factors and doesn't make them worse.

In this country's health-care crisis, there are three crucial issues:

(1) The runaway costs.

(2) The quality of medical treatment.

(3) The problem of more than 35 million uninsured Americans.

In the past few years, more than 100 so-called solutions to the U.S. medical-care crisis have been proposed by the federal government, state governments, and private groups and individuals. More than 30 of these proposals have been considered by Congress.

In nearly every instance, these well-meaning strategies would correct, or improve, the problem of the vast number of uninsured citizens, but by emphasizing that element, they would result in even higher overall costs and a definite deterioration of the quality of medical care.

If a proposal is to be seriously considered, there must be overwhelming evidence that health-care costs will be drastically reduced on a permanent basis, that the quality of America's medical treatment will remain the most efficient in the world, and that every citizen, without exception, be protected against the potential financial disaster of a serious illness.

Here's my Common-Sense Solution that will accomplish each of these goals.

A detailed explanation of this proposal will demonstrate that total costs can be cut almost in half, that most families will be paying less directly out of their pockets than they currently do, that the quality of care will not be diminished and that no one will face financial ruin to cover medical expenses.

The first step is to completely abandon the present system—a system dominated by third-party players and flawed by the misconception that "free" health care is a basic right that is guaranteed.

All state and federal government health programs, including Medicare and Medicaid, would be abolished. There would be no private medical insurance policies or company self-insured programs. Businesses in the U.S. would not be allowed to offer employees any general health-insurance plan as a fringe benefit. These steps will eliminate the need for any third-party players in the country's health-care system.

Now for the details of the "Common-Sense Solution." It is a relatively simple and very efficient plan, consisting of two parts.

First, all Americans, with the exception of the truly poor, would be required to pay out of their pockets all the first part of their health costs, based on their current earnings.

Second, there would be one program, administered by the federal government and funded by taxpayers, that would pay 100 percent of all costs not included in Step One.

The "Common-Sense Solution" is not only an efficient plan that will dramatically reduce costs and improve the quality of health care, it should be an easy program to sell to the American public and government lawmakers, because it will satisfy both those who feel health care should be a free-market vehicle and those who want a national insurance program that covers everyone.

The key to the plan is that it includes both elements. The consumer is put back into the driver's seat and will demand reasonable costs and quality care, while a single health-insurance plan for the more costly episodes will ensure that no one becomes financially devastated by a catastrophic illness. And no one with a medical problem of any type will be denied treatment.

This combination will work! Neither a full free-market plan or an all-inclusive national health-insurance system can succeed by itself. The reason a combination is necessary can be found by studying the breakdown of actual health-care use by individual Americans.

As pointed out earlier, everyone pays dearly for today's faulty health-care system through direct payments to medical professionals, insurance costs, taxes, lower wages and higher prices for goods and services.

Even though we all pay large amounts every year, only a few of us actually have extensive medical treatment in any given year.

According to a recent study by the health-care consulting firm, Milliman & Robertson, only one percent of Americans, or approximately 2.5 million people, incur medical expenses of more than $25,000 in any given year.

Approximately 175 million Americans have little, if any, medical treatment in any given year, according to the National Center for Policy Analysis of Dallas, Texas. Yet, nearly all of these healthy people are paying thousands of dollars each year to protect themselves against the remote possibility of a serious illness.

What a tremendous waste of money!

It's true that many people will have some type of health care in any one year, but most of this is minor and relatively inexpensive.

The Agency for Health-Care Policy and Research, a federal government bureau, has recently released data from an extensive national medical expenditure survey that bears out this fact.

The agency reports that 85.3 percent of all Americans had some type of health care in the year of the survey, but most of this was for dental visits, eyeglasses, routine visits to a doctor, and prescription medicine. Medical expenses of this type could be handled easily by all but a very few of the individuals involved.

The survey showed that in any given year only 14.4 percent of Americans have a hospital confinement, which is the most expensive type of medical care, excluding, of course, nursing home confinement or treatment at chemical-abuse centers. And of all people hospitalized in the year of the survey, four percent of them accounted for 55 percent of all hospital expenses.

There is very little hard evidence on exactly how much medical care each individual in the U.S. requires every year, but studies that have been conducted and the opinions of experts in this field are unanimous that the vast majority has little, if any, treatment and a very small percentage needs extensive care.

J. Patrick Rooney, chairman of the Golden Rule Insurance Co. of Indianapolis, who has studied health expenditures extensively, says, "Only six of every hundred people (six percent) spend more than $3,000 for medical care in any one year."

L. Maynard Oss, president of CORVIEW, Inc., a Minneapolis health-cost management company, who has polled actuaries about expenditures by those who are insured, said only 55 percent of employees or their dependents will collect health benefits in any given year under a typical $200-deductible plan.

That means either 45 percent of these individuals had no medical treatment covered by insurance or the medical care they did have cost less than $200 a year.

Oss says of the 55 percent who collected benefits, 95 percent of them had reimbursements of less than $1,000 in a year. Most of the remaining five percent collected between $1,000 and $5,000.

A survey by Blue Cross & Blue Shield of Ohio of 64,000 of its contract holders shows that 90 percent of them had actual annual medical costs that averaged only $794 each.

The remaining 10 percent had 1989 costs that averaged $10,529 each, which was due primarily to the extremely high expenses of the top one percent, which averaged $56,410 each.

Most health-insurance companies base their premiums on the historical knowledge that only one percent of those insured will file a large claim in any one year.

Under terms of the "Common-Sense Solution," about 90 percent of American households would pay all or most of the costs of their medical care themselves in any one year, while the federal insurance program would cover some or most of the costs of the other 10 percent.

The amount to be paid out-of-pocket would depend on the household's total annual income. A household earning less than $15,000 a year would pay up to a maximum of 10 percent of its income directly before qualifying for federal coverage. So, a household with $8,000 in income would have to pay the first $800 of its costs.

A household with an annual income of between $15,000 and $50,000 would pay 10 percent of the first $15,000 and 12 percent of the balance. This means a household earning $25,000 a year would pay the first $2,700 out-of-pocket, which, in most cases, is less than it is paying today for direct costs, insurance premiums, deductibles and co-payments.

Households with annual incomes between $50,000 and $100,000 would be required to pay 10 percent of the first $15,000, 12 percent of the next $35,000 and 15 percent of everything over $50,000. It would cost a household with an annual income of $75,000 a year a maximum of $9,450 before qualifying for the federal program, which would then pay 100 percent of all additional health-care costs.

There would be a maximum out-of-pocket limit of $19,000 for those with incomes of more than $100,000 a year, so even the wealthiest families would be protected against a catastrophic illness.

(See table on Page 33 for the number of households in various after-tax income categories and the maximum amounts due.)

Keep in mind that these direct costs are for the total household and not for each individual, unless the household consists of only one person.

The important difference between our present system and the "Common-Sense Solution" is that most households have to pay substantial amounts now through insurance premiums, whether they have any medical treatment or not, while this new plan costs only those who actually require health care.

ANNUAL HOUSEHOLD INCOME IN 1991	NUMBER OF HOUSE-HOLDS	MAXIMUM DIRECT MEDICAL EXPENSE
Under $5,000	6,163,524	Zero to $499
$5,000 to $9,999	8,681,777	$500 to $999
$10,000 to $14,999	9,223,373	$1,000 to $1,499
$15,000 to $19,999	9,035,652	$1,500 to $2,099
$20,000 to $24,999	8,345,247	$2,100 to $2,699
$25,000 to $34,999	14,821,094	$2,700 to $3,899
$35,000 to $49,999	16,096,123	$3,900 to $5,699
$50,000 to $99,999	16,584,450	$5,700 to $13,199
More than $100,000	3,293,000	$13,200 to $19,000

Critics of this plan immediately will protest that families couldn't possibly afford to pay 10 percent, 12 percent or 15 percent of their incomes directly for health care. "Unrealistic" and "impossible" they will scream.

The fact is, however, most families today are paying more than that and are facing even higher out-of-pocket expenses in the next several years. The Families USA Foundation, a Washington, D.C.-based non-profit organization, which tracks the actual costs families pay for health care, reports that in 1991 the average U.S. family paid $4,296, or 11.7 percent of its income, in direct costs to support our present health-care system.

The organization reports that families paid 65.7 percent of total medical costs in 1991, while the business community paid the other 34.3 percent.

"Based on current projections," Families USA Foundation says, "average health payments will consume 16.4 percent of average family income by the year 2000. Average health payments by families rose from $1,742 in 1980 to $4,296 in 1991, an increase of 147 percent (average family income climbed by 88 percent during that same period). By the year 2000, average health payments by families are expected to rise to $9,397, an increase of 439 percent over two decades."

The organization says that of the $4,296 in direct costs for the average family, 32 percent of that went for prescription drugs, insurance deductibles and co-payments; 17 percent was spent on out-of-pocket costs for health insurance; 40 percent was in the form of general taxes to support government health programs; 9 percent went for Medicare payroll taxes (from Social Security payments) and 3 percent for Medicare premiums by people over 65.

So, the argument that families couldn't afford the direct costs under the "Common-Sense Solution" is totally incorrect. The main reason most families would be paying far less in out-of-pocket costs is that this new system would result in impressive overall savings.

Because nearly 90 percent of households would not qualify for coverage under the new federal program in any given year, most of the tremendous amount of paperwork now eating up billions of dollars in administrative expenses would be eliminated.

Bookkeeping for people with medical care, who don't qualify for the federal insurance, would involve only a simple bill, made out by the health-care provider and presented to the patient. No records would be forwarded to the administrators of the federal plan. No third-party players would be involved.

Each family or individual would be required to keep track of their out-of-pocket medical costs. When they have reached the maximum amount, the family or individual would present copies of their previously paid bills to the doctor or hospital, etc., who would then authorize future payments to be made by the federal program.

This simplified bookkeeping system should save as much as $200 billion a year in administrative costs by eliminating the staggering expense of today's overly complicated bureaucracy involved in nearly every medical-care case.

A savings of another $200 billion a year would be achieved through the elimination of today's profligate over-utilization of medical services. People who have to pay for services out of their pockets won't take their children to their doctor or hospital for such things as a common cold or a simple case of the flu, and they won't permit extensive testing for minor problems.

(Details of the savings in administrative costs and from the reductions of unnecessary medical care will be outlined in the next chapter.)

Not only would the "Common-Sense Solution" eliminate most of the serious problems in today's flawed system, but it would create an enormous economic boom throughout the country.

This nationwide economic improvement would be the result of lifting off the backs of the U.S. business community its heaviest burden, which is, of course, the staggering costs of providing health insurance for workers.

Businesses are currently paying for nearly 30 percent of all health-care costs, which in 1993 will cost companies $262.5 billion. That's considerably more than the total net profit of all U.S. businesses. Total net profit of all businesses in the country in 1992 was only $250 billion, according to U.S. government statistics.

What would happen if $262.5 billion was pumped back into the business community? The results would be flabbergasting: Millions of new jobs, major expansions by most companies, vast improvement in the ability to compete in the international marketplace, lower prices for goods and services, higher wages for workers, and even larger tax revenues for governments without the need for tax increases.

Under our current medical-care system, companies can deduct the cost of health care from their income taxes. If they have no medical costs, about $90 billion of the $262.5 billion savings would flow to federal and state governments in additional tax revenue.

The overall impact of removing the health-insurance burden from businesses is almost unbelievable.

All businesses would benefit from the "Common-Sense Solution," but the biggest gainers will be the workers at financially troubled companies (and there are many of them), where meeting a payroll is an ever-occurring nightmare.

The large and steady infusion of cash that will result could be the difference between survival and bankruptcy for a large number of struggling businesses. Today, if a company is losing money it doesn't have to pay state or federal income taxes, but there's no relief from stiff and regular payments for health insurance for workers. And the amounts are substantial.

The average annual cost for health-insurance coverage for one worker, including dependents, is now about $5,000 a year with more than 70 percent paid by the company. This compares with only $1,092 in 1980.

The U.S. Chamber of Commerce, after a survey of 1,000 member firms in 1990, said that the $231-per-worker increase that year in health-insurance premium costs was only $29 less than the total of $260 spent per employee for both health and life insurance in 1969.

Unless the present system is drastically changed, costs for health insurance for U.S. workers are expected to increase at a rate of more than 12 percent a year between 1993 and the year 2000, which means the average cost will climb from $5,000 annually per worker with dependent coverage to more than $11,000 by the turn of the century.

Elimination of company health costs will benefit everyone, including consumers, who would see meaningful price reductions, especially for expensive items such as homes, autos, appliances, etc.

A 1992 study by the University of Michigan Transportation Research Institute showed that health-care costs added an average of $1,086 to each U.S.-built automobile. This is 131 percent more than Japanese auto manufacturers pay per auto for health insurance.

In 1991, General Motors Corp. paid $3.4 billion for health care for its 1.9 million employees, dependents and retirees, which is more than the company spent for all the steel used in its autos that year. In 1991, Chrysler Corp. reported that 17 percent of its total payroll costs went to provide health care for its workers.

It's unrealistic to think all the savings would be used to reduce prices, but no matter how the savings are used, the biggest beneficiaries will be workers and consumers.

There also are several peripheral problems that will be ended with the "Common-Sense Solution."

People who today can't qualify for health insurance because of a pre-existing illness will be eligible as everyone else for the benefits offered under the federal coverage.

Workers who hesitate to change jobs because of the fear of losing their health-insurance coverage will have the freedom to accept a new position without medical care being a factor. They won't have to keep a job they hate just because the company has a generous health program.

And people on welfare who hesitate getting back into the job market for fear of losing coverage under generous government medical programs won't have that dilemma.

In the past few years, about eight of every 10 labor strikes in the U.S. have been over health insurance issues.

Without the frequent squabbles over how much workers have to pay for their share of health insurance premiums and how extensive the coverage should be, there will be a much more harmonious relationship between labor unions and management.

Probably the most dramatic change that will result from the "Common-Sense Solution" will be the enormous improvement in government budgets, especially at state and local levels.

In 1993, governments at all levels will be using $423 billion of taxpayer revenues to pay for all types of health costs, including Medicare, Medicaid, veterans and military costs, and other programs, including the expense of providing health care for 17.5 million public employees.

As previously pointed out, there will be about $90 billion in new income tax revenues pouring into government treasuries as the result of companies not being able to deduct as expenses the $262.5 billion they are now paying for workers' medical care.

But that's only part of the story. State and local governments will have no expenses under the "Common-Sense Solution."

Today, according to the U.S. General Accounting Office, state and local governments are spending an average of 20 percent of their total budgets on health care, primarily the state share of Medicaid and health-insurance coverage for the 15 million people employed by cities, towns, counties, school districts and the states.

That amounts to a staggering $126.7 billion, more than enough to solve all the budget problems of state and local governments.

Although the federal government's share of health costs is now $302 billion, when you add the billions of dollars to the U.S. Treasury in new income-tax revenues from businesses that no longer will have health-care deductions and subtract the $12.9 billion in expenses for providing health insurance for the millions of federal employees, the balance is more than enough to fund the program under the "Common-Sense Solution" without any new taxes.

Tremendous Cost Savings

3

Savings in health-care costs under the "Common-Sense Solution" will be staggering. More than $420 billion a year can be slashed from the estimated 1993 total of $906.3 billion, a reduction that most people will find unbelievable.

Although it is impossible to document every dollar of savings, it is not difficult to show substantial amounts can be saved by eliminating much of today's mountains of bureaucratic paperwork, by vastly reducing unnecessary and ineffective medical care, and by shutting the doors that lead to fraud and abuse in our current system.

More than $210 billion in superfluous administration costs could be saved annually within one or two years of implementing the "Common-Sense Solution." An even quicker savings will result from drastically reducing unneeded medical care once families start paying the first part of their costs directly out of their pockets. An estimated $172 billion a year will be saved when individuals discover that their health care isn't "free."

This new plan won't eliminate all the fraud and abuse involved in delivering medical services, but with no insurance programs, Medicaid or Medicare, it is conceivable the amount easily could be cut in half, saving about $45 billion a year.

There would be other savings with this new plan, but they aren't significant compared with the savings made possible by lowering administration costs ($210 billion), reducing unnecessary medical services ($172 billion) and putting the brakes on fraud ($45 billion).

The total annual savings of $427 billion will be challenged, of course, by critics of the "Common-Sense Solution," because these savings are only estimates. They are, however, carefully studied estimates; even so, they could be off by 10 to 20 percent in either direction.

The important thing to remember, though, is that this plan definitely will reduce overall costs dramatically, while nearly all of the other suggested reforms floating around the country involve even higher expenditures than currently being spent in today's flawed system.

To better understand how the "Common-Sense Solution" savings were calculated, let's look closely at each of the three main areas where money is currently wasted, starting with administrative costs.

Health-care experts generally agree that about 30 to 40 percent of today's total costs are due to the extremely heavy load of paperwork at all levels. Much of this load falls on the shoulders of overworked doctors and hospital staffs, but there is a tremendous amount of paper shuffling performed by the nation's 1,250 commercial insurance companies and 73 Blue Cross/Blue Shield plans, by the thousands of clerks and administrators at businesses that provide health insurance for their workers, and by the hordes of third-party players, who futilely attempt to put a lid on soaring costs.

The 30-to-40-percent estimate of administration costs translates into $272 billion to $363 billion in 1993. Let's assume the cost is $300 billion. There always will be some paperwork expense in providing health care under any program, but the "Common-Sense Solution" should trim these costs by about 70 percent.

This 70 percent is not just a wild guess. It is based on a careful analysis of how today's medical costs are broken down (see table on Page 47). There will be two areas where costs can be eliminated entirely. These involve the $64.6 billion being spent in 1993 on administration, profits and overhead for providing private insurance through both commercial insurance companies and self-insurance programs at many large businesses, plus the $15.3 billion now being spent on various third-party administrators.

The elimination of private insurance and the meddling influence of third-party players not only will save almost $80 billion a year, but it will help to vastly improve the quality of medical care.

Is this $80 billion savings an exaggeration? Not if you look at how today's health care is paid. According to various government agencies and several private groups, the private insurance share of 1993 total costs will be $316.2 billion. The $80 billion savings represents about 25 percent of total insurance expenditures.

The 25 percent figure is far less than many groups attribute to administration and other overhead costs involving health insurance. One group, Citizens Fund, claims that commercial health insurers are spending 37.2 percent on administration, marketing and other overhead costs.

Citizens Fund, a research affiliate of the non-profit consumer advocacy organization, Citizen Action, reported in the May 30, 1992, issue of *Medical Benefits* magazine, that commercial insurance spending for administration and other overhead increased by 122 percent between 1981 and 1990, while benefits delivered increased by only 83 percent, which means that administrative spending soared 50 percent faster than benefits paid.

1993 U.S. HEALTH-CARE COSTS

Hospitals---------------------------	$343.1 billion
Physicians-------------------------	$168.2 billion
Nursing homes-------------------	$ 73.4 billion
Drugs and other durables------	$ 65.6 billion
Insurance profits & overhead-	$ 64.6 billion
Optometrists & chiropractors	$ 42.3 billion
Dental services ------------------	$ 41.4 billion
Government public health ----	$ 24.5 billion
Third-party administrators --	$ 15.3 billion
Medical research ----------------	$ 15.1 billion
Other personal health care ---	$ 14.6 billion
Vision products-------------------	$ 14.4 billion
Construction ---------------------	$ 12.0 billion
Home health care ---------------	$ 11.8 billion
TOTALS:	**$906.3 billion**

(These estimates are based on statistics from the U.S. Health Care Financing Administration.)

Citizens Fund claims that one-third of the huge increase in the cost of insurance premiums over the past dozen years was the result of increased administrative expenses.

The research organization says that at least $830 is wasted each year on administrative and overhead costs for a typical family-coverage plan under employer-provided insurance. It claims the cost is even higher for those who don't qualify for company coverage and have to buy their own insurance.

The Health Insurance Association of America disputes the 37.2 percent cost for administration and overhead cited by Citizens Fund, and most other government and private researchers estimate these expenses for insurance at between 20 and 30 percent.

Why does it cost so much to administer insurance programs? Everyone refers to the amount of paper shuffling, but what they are really talking about is the tremendous cost of paying employees to perform these tasks. The *New England Journal of Medicine* reported recently that one insurance company, Blue Cross/Blue Shield of Massachusetts, has 6,682 fulltime workers to provide services for 2.7 million subscribers. That's a larger number of employees than the Canadian government has to administer its national health plan for all of the country's 26.6 million citizens.

While an $80 billion savings resulting from eliminating private insurance and the role of third-party players is impressive, an even larger savings is likely with a less complicated plan for providing treatment at the nation's hospitals.

Again, the waste is centered on the number of employees who spend all or most of their time on paperwork instead of caring for patients. Even though there are fewer hospitals in the U.S. today than a quarter of a century ago, and services have been reduced through improvements in medical procedures, the number of hospital workers has soared. The increase in employment obviously is not because of patient needs. According to the American Hospital Association and the U.S. Health Care Financing Administration, the number of patient hospital days in the U.S. has dropped by 28 percent in the last decade.

There are now 4,980,000 employees working in the country's more than 6,000 hospitals, compared with only 2,690,000 in 1970, an unbelievable increase of 85 percent. Nearly all of this gain is because of the need to fulfill the growing demand for employees to handle paperwork.

Experts attribute 40 to 50 percent of all hospital costs to complying with the various rules and regulations from insurance companies, government bureaucrats and other third-party players. This is probably a conservative estimate when you realize that nearly all of the increase in employment is from added record-keepers and the fact that most nurses now devote about half of their time filling out the multitude of required forms.

Compared with other industrialized countries, the United States far exceeds them in the number of hospital personnel per occupied bed. A 1990 study by the Organization for Economic Cooperation and Development of 23 industrialized countries showed that the U.S. had two-to-four times more hospital workers than most other nations. The study showed that hospitals in the U.S. had an average of 3.35 employees per occupied bed compared with only .79 in Japan, .85 in Austria, 1.09 in France, 1.48 in Germany and Turkey. The U.S. uses much of this huge hospital manpower for administrative purposes.

In another survey of hospitals throughout this country, it was discovered that the average hospital bill today contains more than 50 individual charges, ranging from significant items to a single aspirin or a Kleenex tissue. The average cost of compiling a hospital bill is $120, the survey showed.

During 1993, Americans will be paying hospitals a total of $343.1 billion. If only 40 percent of that is attributed to administration and overhead, it amounts to a whopping $137.2 billion. By eliminating most of the unnecessary paperwork, the "Common-Sense Solution" should easily reduce administrative and overhead costs by 60 percent, for a savings of more than $82 billion.

A third area for huge savings can be found in physicians' offices, where the increase in paperwork is similar to that found in hospitals. Several decades ago when there were no third-party players in the medical field, a physician would keep a brief clinical record of each patient, and the doctor's secretary would type out a bill to be sent to the patient. Today every time a patient visits a doctor, it generates from seven to 10 pieces of paper.

A recent survey of physicians 55 and older by Merritt, Hawkins & Associates, a search firm, shows that most doctors claim they now spend about 20 hours a week on paperwork, including clinical records and various forms for insurers and government agencies, compared with only one to two hours in the early years of their practice.

This huge increase in time spent on paperwork is one of the reasons for the larger number of physicians in the U.S., and is the main reason for the staggering increase in the number of office workers in doctors' offices.

There are now more than 600,000 physicians in the U.S., according to the American Medical Association, which figures out to 240 physicians per 100,000 population. In 1970 there were 148 physicians for each 100,000. That's a gain of 62 percent, which is relatively small compared to the enormous increase in the number of office workers during the same period. In 1970 there were 477,000 people working in physicians' offices throughout the country. Today there are 1,339,000 employed in those offices, a gain of 181 percent.

As in hospitals, the tremendous increase of workers in physicians' offices is due almost entirely to the growing burden of producing records for insurers, government bureaucrats, other third-party players and for the doctors' attorneys in the event of malpractice lawsuits.

Bureaucrats and other third parties acknowledge that regulation of the medical industry might generate additional costs, but they claim a large amount of money will be saved by their intensive supervision.

Unfortunately, the facts show that much more money is wasted on this over-regulation than is saved. In 1990, for instance, the inspector general of the U.S. Health and Human Services Department reported that the federal government paid several utilization companies $13.3 million to examine 500,000 Medicare cataract operations. The careful examination ended up saving $1.4 million in what was determined to be "possible unnecessary surgery." That means taxpayers spent $13.3 million to save $1.4 million in medical costs. And this isn't an isolated example.

The total number of dollars going to physicians during 1993 will reach $168.2 billion. A doctor's pre-tax income now averages $164,000 annually, which means that $98.5 billion of the total goes for physician salaries and taxes. The remaining $69.7 billion is for overhead, most of it directly linked to paperwork.

If total overhead can be cut in half through the "Common-Sense Solution," the savings will amount to almost $35 billion.

So if $80 billion can be saved through eliminating insurance administration and overhead, $82 billion can be saved by reducing paperwork in hospitals and another $35 billion in the offices of physicians, this amounts to a total of $197 billion. Only another $13 billion has to be saved in administrative costs at all other health-care providers—nursing homes, dentists, chiropractors, and other professionals—to meet the goal of $210 billion.

Now let's look at the possible savings from reducing the amount of unnecessary health care.

Dozens of individuals and organizations have attempted in recent years to analyze the problem of unneeded medical care and to arrive at the amount of money wasted. The experts agree the amount is substantial, but their estimates vary considerably.

Perhaps the most exhaustive nationwide study of the problem was conducted in 1991 by Milliman & Robertson, Inc., a provider of actuarial and consulting services to the health-care industry. After analyzing thousands of medical-chart reviews on patients, Milliman & Robertson researchers concluded that "53 percent of our current health-care costs are medically unnecessary."

Another high estimate comes from CORVIEW, Inc., a Minneapolis-based medical management company, which recently stated, "Most clinicians will agree that 75 to 80 percent of physician office calls, particularly initial calls, are unnecessary from a strict medical point of view."

The vast majority of experts who have studied the problem agree the amount wasted on unnecessary and ineffective medical services is at least one-third of the nation's total health-care costs, which means Americans are wasting a whopping $300 billion this year.

Undoubtedly no system would completely eliminate all unneeded medical care, but it's conceivable the "Common-Sense Solution" would chop off more than half the waste, because consumers would be in direct control of what they pay health-care providers.

Regardless of the goods or services involved, consumers are naturally careless when they don't pay directly for them. If groceries were purchased in the manner health-care is paid for today, the waste would be horrendous. If Americans had an insurance program to cover the cost of purchasing automobiles, most of them would be driving luxury cars and would be trading them every year.

It's a human tendency to be exceedingly careful when you have to pay directly out of your pocket for something, and to be careless when a purchase doesn't affect your pocketbook immediately.

Credit-card abuse is an example of what happens when a person can buy a product or service without paying at the time of the purchase. Somehow a consumer feels the price is not so important when cash is not required.

Congress discovered this phenomenon when its plan for withholding income taxes proved successful. Most Americans would revolt if they had to shell out thousands of dollars in cash at the end of the year for their income taxes, but they are complacent when the system takes away a much smaller amount out of each paycheck before they even see the money.

Although many people blame doctors and hospitals for encouraging patients to accept services that are not medically necessary, most of the blame today rests with patients and their families who have little concern about the cost when most of it is paid by insurance companies or the government.

Two touchy areas of wasteful—and extremely costly—medical care concern premature newborn babies who have practically no chance of survival, and elderly patients only days away from certain death.

An article in the Feb. 26, 1992, edition of the *Wall Street Journal,* tells of a typical case—the futile efforts to prolong the life of a terminally-ill 90-year-old patient. The man was suffering from severe bilateral pneumonia, a fractured hip, and gradual respiratory, kidney and heart failure. His doctors at New York City's St. Luke's-Roosevelt Hospital were certain death was imminent, but they still proceeded with costly aggressive care. Despite the respirator, heart monitor, feeding tubes, antibiotics, X-rays, blood tests and sedatives, the patient died within a few days, but the medical costs for those final days of care amounted to $93,111.

The *Journal* article detailed some of the costly procedures: "On admission to the intensive-care unit, the patient had a Swan Ganz catheter inserted into his pulmonary artery to record cardiac output and an arterial line to monitor blood pressure (a $313 procedure). Before he died, he had 70 arterial blood gas analyses and 156 other blood tests ($22 to $42 each), 38 X-rays ($70 to $310 each), a cardiac ultra-sound ($230), and 13 blood transfusions ($90 each)."

Most of the cost of this treatment was covered by Medicare, of course.

The *Journal* article also reported that similar aggressive treatment was being performed on an irreversibly brain-damaged patient in a nearby bed. This patient received 50 blood tests, 16 X-rays, a CT scan, two abdominal ultrasounds, more than a dozen bacterial cultures and five blood transfusions before she died after 18 days.

The *Journal* correctly points out that for hopelessly ill patients, this type of care is "at best marginally useless."

More than 14 percent of total health-care costs, or about $130 billion, is spent each year treating patients in the final days before their deaths. Some of this care is warranted, especially in the cases of younger patients with at least some chances of survival, but much of it is unnecessary. As long as the patients or their families aren't responsible for paying any of the enormous amounts, there is little incentive to use good judgment in deciding who should receive aggressive care.

A 1992 survey of patients by the American Medical Association showed that 63 percent of those interviewed said they never inquired about the cost of the medical services involved before treatment.

And, too often, when a patient brings up the subject of costs, the answer is, "Don't worry, your insurance will take care of it."

Much of the attention paid to unnecessary medical care is centered on very expensive treatment, such as the care cited in the *Journal* article or heart by-pass surgery and cesarean sections, and while these major services are important areas to study, the main waste today is in treatment of ailments that normally go away with or without professional help.

Most of the visits to physicians' offices, clinics and hospital emergency rooms are for common illnesses such as the common cold, influenza, sore throats, back pain, and stomach aches. Nearly all of these problems fall into this category: "Without treatment it will go away in a week, but if you see a doctor it will be cured in seven days."

When health insurance covers all or most of the cost of an illness, it's natural for people to seek professional care, but when they have to pay directly out of their pockets, these same people will be very cautious about spending money on minor illnesses.

A good example of how "free" medical care encourages unnecessary visits to doctors and hospitals is found in the country's Medical Assistance program, the most generous in the Medicaid system. It provides care to people on welfare and other low-income families and normally involves no payment from the patients, most of whom are single mothers and their children. The joint federal-state government program is operated by the states.

The cost of the Medicaid program has exploded in the past five years, and is now rising at a staggering rate of 30 percent a year, according to a 1992 study by the Kaiser Family Foundation.

The foundation reported that costs for Medicaid in 1992 reached $120 billion, up from only $51.6 billion in 1988.

Last year in Minnesota, there were 423,000 people enrolled in the Medical Assistance program, and the state Department of Human Services processed more than 13 million claims, which means that each person had an average of 30 visits to doctors and hospitals or trips to the drug store for medicine in a single year.

In an attempt to hold down the soaring costs of the Medical Assistance program, government Medicaid bureaucrats, instead of recognizing that most of the services provided are unnecessary, have placed limits on what they will pay for the professional treatment.

Doctors claim that these Medicaid price limits mean they have to accept about half their normal charges for treating these patients, and, consequently, many doctors are refusing to accept new patients on Medical Assistance.

The price limits have forced many Medicaid patients to seek treatment at hospital emergency rooms, instead of looking for a physician that will accept them.

During the winter of 1992, six Chicago-area hospitals were forced to turn away ambulances with ill people in them because their emergency rooms were jammed full, mostly with patients with colds or the flu. Dr. David Meyers, director of the emergency room at Resurrection Hospital in Chicago, said his hospital was turning away patients periodically for more than two months, primarily due to the city's flu outbreak.

Since the beginning of Medicaid price controls, hospital emergency rooms throughout the country have seen their patient loads nearly double, and administrators admit that most emergency-room visits are of a non-emergency nature.

Seeking medical treatment for minor illnesses isn't limited to people on Medicaid. Several studies show that people with any type of health insurance are more than twice as likely to seek professional care than those without coverage.

Requiring everyone to pay the first part of their medical care out of their pockets not only would dramatically cut down unnecessary visits, but it would encourage people to shop around for quality treatment at the lowest possible price.

Knowledgeable people already know that prices for medical treatment vary considerably, but most Americans today simply accept whatever is offered without "shopping around."

Karolina Wilson, a registered nurse in Kalamazoo, Mich., knows firsthand the benefits of "shopping around."

In a May 12, 1992, column in the *Kalamazoo Gazette*, she told how beneficial it can be to check medical prices in the same manner a careful consumer shops for a new television set.

Wilson had been to her physician for an annual checkup and was told she needed an ultrasound examination of her ovaries. She discovered that the hospital recommended by her doctor would charge her $291 for the examination. She checked by phone with eight other places that offered the same ultrasound test and learned the cost was different at each place. She selected a radiology laboratory that charged only $120, saving her the tidy sum of $171.

Wilson said, "What I did was something that anyone can do. It really irritates me that the health-care consumer is not educated about options. Too many patients see the physicians as too intimidating and don't question what they are told to do. Sometimes the patient or the doctor doesn't have the time to pursue options, but when we do have the time, we really should shop around. When we don't, it costs all of us."

Karolina Wilson's intelligent attitude would spread throughout the country if consumers had to pay the first part of their medical costs directly. That's the way human beings are.

It's only common sense to believe that by paying directly for health care, consumers wouldn't seek unnecessary professional care for minor ailments and they would shop around for the best possible price for treatment that is needed. They also would be much more aggressive in their relationships with health-care providers, challenging suggestions for various tests and procedures that might be unnecessary.

Because insurers and government agencies now pay most of the costs, physicians are much more likely to suggest their patients undergo expensive testing "just to make sure" and to protect doctors from possible malpractice suits.

Even more wasteful is the growing trend of specialists to repeat medical tests that have already been performed. When a patient is transferred from one hospital to another where there are more competent specialists, it is common to start fresh with the various diagnostic testing at tremendous unnecessary costs rather than to accept the medical history from the previous hospital.

The Federal Centers for Disease Control estimates that more than $50 billion a year is wasted on needless medical tests. The American Medical Association says that a recent survey showed that 80 percent of physicians order more tests than necessary. As medical technology improves, there are many more tests available than just a few years ago. It is now possible, for example, to conduct more than 900 different tests on a patient's blood.

There's little doubt that if individuals were paying directly for these tests, the number would be reduced drastically, and billions of dollars would be saved.

The third area of considerable savings if the "Common Sense Solution" was adopted is in today's rampant fraud and abuse in medical care. Although most health-care providers and patients are honest, even a small number of crooks can account for a large loss of precious medical funds.

The U.S. General Accounting Office, the National Health Care Anti-Fraud Association, several insurance companies and many other groups and individuals agree that at least 10 percent of today's medical costs is drained off through fraud and abuse. In 1993 that means about $90 billion is being wasted.

It's quite apparent that as the present medical system becomes more complicated, the amount of fraud and abuse soars. Nearly everyone involved in health care is getting more concerned about the growing problem, especially the federal government, insurers and the American Medical Association.

About 40 percent of health insurance companies have started anti-fraud programs in the past few years, according to the Health Insurance Association, a Washington, D.C., trade group. The Federal Bureau of Investigation (FBI) has added 50 agents to the crew of 46 already assigned to health-care fraud. About 125 assistant U.S. attorneys are currently assigned to the program throughout the country with special anti-fraud units established in the 12 cities where the problem is most acute. These cities are Los Angeles, Baltimore, Chicago, Dallas, Detroit, Las Vegas, Miami, New York, New Orleans, Philadelphia, Newark and Charlotte, N.C.

Congress and federal bureaucrats are beginning to regard medical fraud as a very serious problem. The inspector general's office of the U.S. Health and Human Services Department has endorsed a new bill that will crack down hard on health-care fraud. The bill would require prison terms of up to 10 years and fines up to $250,000 for physicians, pharmacists, hospitals and medical-equipment suppliers who are found guilty of health-care fraud.

The new legislation also would allow the government to seize any profits from health-care fraud, and it would hold the hospital responsible for any fraudulent acts of one of its physicians. The bill would add several hundred new federal investigators to the growing number already devoting fulltime to medical fraud.

The American Medical Association says it has become more "militant" about health-care fraud by a very small percentage of the nation's doctors, but it strongly opposes the overly stringent bill being considered by Congress.

No system will reduce fraud and abuse to a zero amount, but the current problem is due mostly to the fact that third parties, instead of patients themselves, are paying the bills.

Complicated billing systems of insurers and government agencies cause most of today's fraud and abuse. The problem is especially acute at hospitals, where numerous outside audits have shown an extraordinary number of overcharges, many accidental and an unknown number deliberate.

If you've ever received a billing from a hospital, you can appreciate how complicated these statements are, and you probably won't be surprised to learn that many contain errors.

The fact that most of the hospital errors are overcharges rather than undercharges indicates that the problem is more than just carelessness. *Hospital Magazine*, an industry trade publication, estimates that 96 percent of all hospital bills contain overcharges, an amount that is higher than most estimates, but lower than some. The General Accounting Office, an arm of the U.S. Congress, reviewed patient records at four Los Angeles-area hospitals recently and discovered that 99 percent of the cases audited contained overcharges. One health insurance company reported that its audits of hospital bills of more than $10,000 showed an average overcharge of $955.

Problems in hospital billings are due not so much to dishonesty as to desperation. Plagued by complicated rules, regulations and cost controls by third parties, most U.S. hospitals are struggling to survive, and they have to take desperate measures to stay alive. According to a May 1992 study by Health Care Investment Analysts, nearly one of every five U.S. hospitals is financially "distressed." Most hospitals are non-profit organizations, and it's unfair to accuse them of attempting to defraud the public. Even for-profit hospitals are having financial difficulties due to unreasonable outside interference with their main function of providing medical care to patients.

A good example of the complex regulations interfering with efficient hospital billing is the Medicare program. Nearly 40 percent of hospital admissions today are Medicare patients (those 65 and over). The federal Medicare statute is 142 pages long. There are another 400 pages of regulations and 11,000 pages of instructions.

If hospital bills were less complicated and sent directly to the patient, who would be responsible for paying some or all of the charges, it's logical the number of overcharges would be significantly reduced.

Overcharges by health-care providers is only one area where fraud and abuse are involved. There are organized criminal rings routinely ripping off insurance companies and especially the Medicaid and Medicare programs through prescription-drug scams. Crooked sales people in many areas of the country are selling unneeded medical equipment to older people in their homes and billing the federal government or other insurers. And there is a growing amount of insurance abuse at many psychiatric clinics and chemical dependency treatment centers.

Law-enforcement agencies are beginning to regard medical fraud as an increasingly serious problem. In June 1992, more than 1,000 FBI agents and 120 other federal officers conducted a massive nationwide crackdown on prescription drug fraud, arresting more than 100 people in a single day, including 82 pharmacists. The sweep involved arrests in 50 cities.

Those arrested were charged with a variety of offenses, including filling prescriptions with generic drugs but billing insurance companies and Medicaid for much more expensive brand-name products. Some of the pharmacists were accused of charging insurers several times for the same prescription and charging for prescriptions that were never written or filled.

One of the more common drug scams in the federal crackdown involved welfare recipients eligible for Medicaid benefits. They would visit a doctor, who was in on the fraud, and receive a prescription for an expensive drug. The physician would charge Medicaid for a complete physical exam and other tests that were never conducted. The "patient" would take the prescription to a pharmacist, who also was part of the scheme, and instead of the expensive drug, a cheap generic drug was substituted. The pharmacist would bill Medicaid, however, for the expensive drug. The "patient" would then sell the drug on the street to another conspirator, who then would sell the drug back to the same pharmacist that filled the prescription. Federal officers said this type of organized fraud is becoming common throughout the country.

Fraud and abuse are part of any human activity, but by removing insurance companies entirely and minimizing the role of government in the payment of medical expenses, the $90-billion annual cost easily could be cut in half, saving another $45 billion.

Add that $45 billion to the $210 billion that could be saved by reducing superfluous paperwork and the $172 billion in the reduction of unnecessary medical treatment, and the "Common-Sense Solution" could cut current health-care costs almost in half.

No other proposed reform of the country's medical-care system even comes close to saving that amount.

How About the Poor?

4

Before fully understanding the details of the "Common-Sense Solution," many people are likely to criticize the plan as being unaffordable for a large number of Americans, especially those who are unemployed or working at lowly paid jobs.

For example, critics will be quick to point out that a mother on welfare supporting three small children can barely raise the cash for rent, food and clothing, much less pay $600 for medical care. They'll also claim that a family struggling along with $12,000 in annual income would have a difficult time coming up with $1,200 of their own cash to pay medical bills.

But the "Common-Sense Solution" has been carefully designed so that poor people would be reimbursed for all or most of their out-of-pocket medical costs, and 95 percent of other Americans would be paying less in direct payments than they are under the current system.

With very few exceptions, the only people who would be paying more under this system would be a handful of super-wealthy families, facing a maximum of $19,000 a year in direct payments. Even the wealthy, however, would be protected against the enormous cost of a catastrophic illness.

How will the poor be protected under the new plan?

Let's look first at welfare recipients who, under Medicaid, have the most generous insurance plan in existence today. The medical-assistance program, funded jointly by state and federal governments, offers first-dollar coverage to more than 27 million people who are in various welfare programs.

Because there is no shared expense in the welfare medical plan, there has been a tremendous amount of over-utilization of medical services, and costs have been soaring in recent years at an annual rate of more than 30 percent.

Taxpayers today are spending more on health care for the poor than they are for the combined total of cash welfare payments, food stamps, rent-and-utility assistance, child nutrition, the Supplemental Security Income program, and the earned-income tax credit for the working poor.

If Medicaid is eliminated and welfare recipients are responsible for medical costs equal to 10 percent of their cash benefits each year, the over-utilization will be significantly reduced and total costs will be cut tremendously. But where will welfare recipients find the money to pay anything out-of-pocket?

Benefits paid to people on the country's largest welfare program, Aid to Families with Dependent Children (AFDC), vary from state to state, but to show how the new plan will work, let's use Wisconsin as an example. Wisconsin pays a monthly cash benefit of $517 for a single mother with two children, slightly higher than the average of all states.

The annual cash payment to this family is $6,204 a year, which means that under the "Common-Sense Solution" the family would pay the first $620 of medical care out-of-pocket. The amount the family receives in food stamps, rent assistance and other non-cash benefits is not included in the medical-cost formula.

Under the new system, welfare households throughout the country will receive an additional $65 per month to make up for the loss of the current medical-assistance program. The $65 per month would be more than welfare recipients need to pay for their new direct medical costs in nearly all states. If any of the additional $780 annual cash payment was not needed for medical expenses, the family could use the money for any purpose it wanted.

By increasing the monthly cash benefit, welfare recipients not only could afford their share of health-care costs, but they would be less likely to overuse medical services, and the exorbitant cost of today's health-care system for the poor would be reduced significantly.

The increased payments to all welfare recipients will total only about $7.8 billion a year, while the savings involved in eliminating all Medicaid benefits would exceed $144 billion annually.

Now, let's examine an even bigger problem—working people with incomes insufficient to meet all their needs. These are the people that today make up the largest share of those with no health-care insurance. They have no medical insurance because they work for small companies that don't offer this fringe benefit or they are self-employed. Most of these people can't afford the $3,000 to $5,000 annual premiums for private family coverage.

The 35 million Americans without health insurance is the problem with the highest priority among those who are seeking solutions to the present medical-cost crisis.

The "Common-Sense Solution" is the only plan that will cover these people, along with all other Americans, without increasing total health-care costs.

Low-income workers will be required to pay up-front medical costs along with all other citizens, but those with family incomes of $12,000 a year or less will receive a tax credit for most of their out-of-pocket expenditures.

As an example, let's look at a married couple with two children who earn $12,000 a year and have out-of-pocket medical costs of $800 in a calendar year. When filing their federal income tax form that year, they list the $800 expense, not as a deduction but as a credit, and they will receive 80 percent of the $800, or $640, in addition to any other refund they might have coming. This means that the family actually had only $160 in out-of-pocket expenses for medical care.

Let's say this same family had direct medical expenses of $1,200 for the year, the maximum amount a family with an annual income of $12,000 would be required to pay. The refund they would receive from the federal government would be $960, or 80 percent of the amount they paid, meaning their out-of-pocket expense for the year would be only $240.

Every household with an annual income of $12,000 or less would be eligible to receive the medical-expense tax-credit refund even if no income taxes were owed.

This plan for low-income families will accomplish two important goals. First, it would offer quality medical care at an affordable cost to people who are excluded today from the system. Second, because they would be required to pay the first part of their medical costs when incurred and get their refund later, there is an incentive to use the health-care system carefully.

How about low-income families who are unable to come up with the cash to cover medical costs when incurred? They will be able to set up a monthly payment plan with doctors or hospitals, or, as a last resort, the refund check could be claimed by the health-care provider.

There is another group of poor people who do not fit into either of the two previous categories. They are not on welfare and they have little if any income at all. Many of them are homeless or will be in the near future.

These people sometimes need medical care, too, and they will receive it under this new plan without the hassle they face today. Because they have no income, there is no up-front cost for them. They will qualify immediately for the government coverage.

Providing tax credits to the working poor and totally free medical service to the homeless and and other destitute Americans will be expensive, adding about $14 billion a year to medical-care costs. But this new expense will be more than offset by a massive reduction in the current amount of unpaid services by health-care providers.

Most of the delinquent bills on the books of hospitals and physicians' offices today come from patients who are uninsured, especially the working poor, the unemployed and the homeless. These are the people who, under this new plan, will have the ability to pay their medical costs.

Naturally some charges by health-care providers will continue to go unpaid under the new system, but the total amount will be significantly reduced through the tax credits and the federal government coverage.

The most recent data available show that well over $31 billion of medical costs go unpaid each year. The American Hospital Association reports that in 1990, U.S. hospitals provided $17.8 billion of uncompensated care. Physicians report that more than 8 percent of their billings remain unpaid, an amount that totals more than $13.4 billion a year. And this doesn't include the additional billions of unpaid bills at the offices of dentists, optometrists, chiropractors, nursing homes and other health-care providers.

Because the staggering costs of these unpaid medical bills are passed on to other patients and taxpayers, it's safe to assume that any of the new costs under the "Common-Sense Solution" will be far less than the savings involved.

So, if this new plan fully protects families on welfare, those currently without health insurance, and the homeless, how about the 138.7 million workers who today have medical insurance through their employers and the 30 million Americans who currently buy their own insurance?

All of these people will receive medical care of a quality that is equal to, or better than, the care they presently get, with no interference from defiant third parties, and at an out-of-pocket cost that, for nearly all of them, will be less than they are now paying.

A few years ago, most Americans with health insurance paid very little out-of-pocket cash for their medical care. But as costs soared, insurance companies were forced to dramatically increase deductibles and co-payments, while employers demanded that workers start paying part of the premium for their coverage.

Each year these employee contributions, deductibles and co-payments have been increasing, and there is no indication the out-of-pocket costs won't continue to soar for the next several years if radical changes aren't implemented.

According to the February 1992 issue of *Employers' Health Benefits Letter*, 48 percent of U.S. companies have increased the amount of employee contributions for medical insurance during the past three years, while 44 percent increased the cost of deductibles. A poll of 250 companies in Winston-Salem, N.C., by Booke & Co. in 1992 showed that 93 percent of the businesses were planning to raise the employee share of health costs before the year ended.

The average out-of-pocket costs today for people covered by family health insurance is more than $2,000 annually, and the total amount is growing each year by double-digit percentages.

The U.S. Department of Health reports that in 1980 only 5.8 percent of health insurance costs were paid by workers, while today they pay more than 30 percent.

A survey by Hay/Huggins & Co. shows that in 1980 a typical worker contributed only $150 a year toward premiums for health insurance, compared with $1,300 annually in 1990. The survey also showed that in 1980 more than 40 percent of companies paid the full cost of premiums for family health-insurance coverage.

Today more than 90 percent of companies require contributions from employees for family coverage, and it is apparent that within a few years no firm will be paying all costs for health insurance.

General Motors Corp., one of the last major companies in the country to pay 100 percent of health-care costs for employees and retirees, admitted in late 1992 it was considering various proposals to require contributions from workers and retirees. The nation's largest auto manufacturer was planning to start with non-union salaried employees and retirees and then prepare for an expected battle with union leaders in a desperate move to reduce its soaring medical costs.

Even government employees, most of whom in the past enjoyed fully-paid, first-dollar health insurance, now are subject to premium contributions, deductibles, and co-payments.

In 1991 only 10 states didn't require government workers to pay part of their insurance costs.

A survey by the Segal Company of state governments showed that public employees who contributed to their family health insurance coverage paid an average of $1,368 a year in 1991, up 12 percent from the year before. Deductibles, co-payments and other costs were in addition to that amount.

The Public Affairs Institute of New Jersey, studying the impact of out-of-pocket health-insurance expenses of workers in that state for payroll contributions, deductibles and co-payments, discovered that the maximum costs being charged to workers were much higher than suspected.

In 1991 a family of four headed by a worker employed at a public utility faced maximum out-of-pocket expenses of $4,140 annually. It was $3,490 for an insurance company worker with three dependents, $3,321 for a commercial bank employee and $1,800 for a government employee.

Workers throughout the country are discovering that health insurance is a fringe benefit that is no longer "free," and most of them will welcome the "Common-Sense Solution" that will provide better health care at a lower direct cost.

Another large group of Americans who will benefit greatly under this new plan are those 65 and over. Most of these 34.3 million senior citizens are currently "covered" by Medicare, but the federal government program pays only about half of their medical expenses.

Medicare coverage is not only inadequate, it is grossly unfair in its treatment of people with different incomes and net worth. For example, a widow over 65 with very little net worth and monthly income of only $600 from Social Security pays the same Medicare premium as an elderly person with millions of dollars in savings and investments and a very sizable annual income.

They both collect the same benefits, which are much less than those of the typical working person with a standard insurance policy. In fact, elderly families are spending more today directly out-of-pocket than they did in inflation-adjusted dollars before Medicare was started. According to Families USA Foundation, the average elderly family in the U.S. was spending $3,305 annually on health care in 1991 compared with $1,589 in 1961 (in 1991 dollars).

Because Medicare's inadequate protection against the cost of a serious illness, most of the elderly are forced to buy supplemental insurance coverage, often referred to as Medigap policies. Although not as expensive as most health-insurance policies for people under 65, these Medigap plans add a substantial amount to the elderly's out-of-pocket costs. About 80 percent of people covered by Medicare also carry supplemental insurance.

Medicare recipients without Medigap policies must pay a $628 deductible for hospital care plus a co-payment of $78.50 a day after the first three weeks in a skilled nursing facility. There also is a $100 deductible for physicians' services. There is no coverage for most routine medical tests, immunizations, hearing aids or eyeglasses. Even the elderly with Medigap policies in addition to Medicare must pay large amounts for prescription drugs.

A person with Medicare coverage but no supplemental policy faces financial disaster today if a lengthy hospital stay is necessary. A Medicare patient must pay $163 daily after the first 60 days and $326 a day after 150 days.

The U.S. Bureau of Labor Statistics, in a recent survey of consumer spending patterns, pointed out that Americans over 65 spend nearly three times as much out-of-pocket for health care than households headed by people aged 35 to 44.

It's true, of course, that the elderly use medical services much more than younger Americans, but many people over 65 are living on small fixed incomes and simply can't afford current costs for a serious illness.

Under the "Common-Sense Solution," all of the elderly would be protected and most will be paying far less than under the current system.

The elderly widow with a $600-a-month Social Security income, who today could expect to be personally billed more than $34,000 for a seven-month stay in a hospital if she did not have Medigap coverage, would owe a maximum of $720 out-of-pocket under the new plan, and she would get most of that back through the tax-credit plan.

Elderly people who are wealthy would have to pay a substantial amount out-of-pocket, up to a maximum of $19,000 a year, but about 99 percent of those over 65 would pay much less than they currently do.

In addition to having quality medical care available to them at an affordable cost, the nation's elderly would have, under the "Common-

Sense Solution," peace of mind instead of night after night of restless sleep caused by the worry of being trapped in the current system.

In fact, all Americans would have this peace of mind knowing that the new system is not only workable but affordable to everyone.

Big Economic Boost

5

A complete overhaul of the present unworkable health-care system will dramatically lower costs while improving the quality of service, and as a pleasant extra advantage, it will give the country's economy a very badly needed shot-in-the-arm. This economic boost will occur by removing from U.S. businesses the horrendous cost of providing medical care for workers.

In 1993 businesses will be spending an estimated $262.5 billion for employee medical benefits, a projection based on the latest available data from the U.S. Health Care Financing Administration. (See table on Page 85). This includes $196.4 billion for employee health insurance, $41.5 billion in company payments to the Medicare hospital insurance trust fund from Social Security taxes, and $24.6 billion for the medical-cost share of workers compensation.

Although it is not included in official health-care statistics, most companies also are spending sizable amounts on salaries and benefits for those employees who devote all or most of their time handling the complex health-care administrative duties.

Because the total net after-tax profit of all U.S. companies in 1992 was about $250 billion, the savings of $262.5 billion in health-care costs would mean, in effect, that total business profits would more than double once the burden was removed.

With the infusion of such a tremendous amount of additional working capital, most companies would expand vigorously, resulting in millions of new jobs, and giving U.S. businesses a vastly improved ability to compete with foreign firms that today have a tremendous advantage with their lower operating costs.

The business community is well aware of the seriousness of its medical-cost problem, even though most citizens and government officials are not yet ready to recognize it as a severe financial crisis that affects nearly everyone.

U.S. MEDICAL COSTS FOR 1993 ACCORDING TO TYPE OF PAYER

(in billions of dollars)

Businesses-------$262.5	
Employer payments to company health-insurance premiums----------------	$196.4
Employer payments to Medicare hospital insurance trust fund---------------	$ 41.5
Workers compensation medical costs--------	$ 24.6
Individuals-------$316.8	
Employee payments to premiums for company health insurance and individual policies---------------------	$ 70.4
Employee and self-employment payments to Medicare hospital trust fund -------------	$ 40.2
Premiums paid by individuals to Medicare hospital trust fund---------------------------	$ 14.3
Out-of-pocket spending for medical services & prescription drugs--------------	$191.9
Federal government--------$200.3*	
Payments for health insurance for public employees and retirees---------------	$ 12.9
Adjusted Medicare (does not include payments from businesses, individuals and state and local governments)----------	$ 61.3
Medicaid--------------------------------------	$ 83.4
Dept. of Veterans Affairs----------------------	$ 16.1
Dept. of Defense--------------------------------	$ 16.2
Other programs -------------------------------	$ 10.4
State and local governments-----$126.7	
Payments for health insurance for public employees and retirees---------------	$ 36.5
Payments to Medicare hospital insurance trust fund------------------------	$ 5.7
Medicaid---------------------------------------	$ 60.6
Hospital subsidies------------------------------	$ 11.8
Other programs--------------------------------	$ 12.1

*The $200.3 billion represents the amount paid by the federal government for health care from general taxes. Adding Medicare taxes paid by businesses, individuals and state and local governments increases the actual federal share to $302 billion

In a May 1992 survey by the National Federation of Independent Business, the cost of health care was overwhelmingly declared the No.1 problem facing companies today. No other problem, among the 75 examined, was even close.

Nearly all of those surveyed listed the cost of health care the most serious problem facing business, and 61 percent termed it "critical," the most extreme assessment listed in the survey. Even the businesses that do not currently provide health coverage listed it as a serious problem. Workers compensation insurance, which actually is part of the health-care crisis, was listed by those in the survey as the second most serious problem facing businesses today.

Other problems, which were listed far below health care and workers compensation costs, were (in order of seriousness) federal taxes on business income, cash flow, liability insurance costs, Social Security taxes, state taxes on business income, unreasonable government regulations, property taxes and rent costs, and frequent changes in federal tax laws.

Twenty years ago the cost of providing health care for workers was not a serious burden. Today it is a crisis. Tomorrow?

It's obvious that if the soaring costs of health care aren't drastically reduced or eliminated—and soon—businesses will be forced to either drop their insurance programs or shift most of the cost to employees, unless, of course, the federal government forces businesses to provide medical insurance. And that would be an economic disaster.

Businesses are currently providing health insurance for 138.7 million workers and their dependents, or seven of every 10 Americans under the age of 65, according to the Employee Benefits Research Institute.

During the past several years, most U.S. businesses have given high priority to reducing health-care costs and have taken extreme measures to do so, but total expenses continue to soar. Shifting more of the cost to workers, self-insurance programs, and managed-care systems have slowed the increases somewhat, but overall costs have jumped by double-digit percentages year after year.

The futility of these efforts was demonstrated in a 1992 study by the New York firm, Ernst & Young, which retained Louis Harris and Associates to interview corporate benefits officers of the country's 2,500 largest companies.

The study showed that 90 percent of the companies engaged in some degree of cost containment during the three previous years, nearly half of which were described as very comprehensive. Only 21 percent of the companies in the study said the results were "very effective."

Of companies in the study that have adjusted their health-care programs, most report that their average annual per-capita medical costs are only about $100 less than the average of all U.S.

companies. Those companies that feel their medical costs are "out of control" have average annual per worker costs that were only about $150 above the average of all firms.

The Ernst & Young study, plus other evidence, indicate that no matter what steps are taken, medical costs are almost impossible to reduce.

Another 1992 study, this one by the Conference Board, showed that 75 percent of the chief executive officers of the nation's biggest companies feel there is "not a reasonable chance" they will be able to contain health-care costs within the next five years. More than half of the executives believe that government legislation is needed to coordinate public and private health-care plans in order to eliminate more cost shifting to employees.

Although most business leaders in the U.S. are strong believers in the free enterprise system, more and more of them are becoming so disillusioned with the present health-care machinery that they are willing to support a program totally operated by government, i.e., socialized medicine, which has failed in just about every country that has tried it.

Many top executives believe the only other alternative remaining is to abandon their employee health coverage.

If companies suddenly stopped providing medical coverage for employees before a workable health-care system is adopted in this country, the number of Americans with no insurance would soar to the point where our present system would collapse.

Something drastic has to be done before this occurs.

The "Common-Sense Solution" is the only system that would prevent the pending disaster, because it would lower total health-care costs without reducing the quality of care or access to it. A national health system handled entirely by the government would merely switch business costs from direct payments to even higher expenses through taxes. Most other "reforms" under consideration place the bulk of the additional costs on the backs of businesses.

The present system that ties health insurance primarily to employment is unworkable and has been filled with flaws since it was started back in the mid-1930s. It is inefficient and unfair, and along with Medicare and Medicaid, is responsible for today's uncontrollable costs.

Companies of all sizes are suffering from unaffordable health-care costs, but small firms are especially vulnerable. John Galles, president of National Small Business United, claims that small businesses pay on average about 40 percent more than large companies for the same type of medical insurance, and because 86 percent of all U.S. businesses have fewer than 20 employees, the problem is worse than most people recognize.

The government is contributing immensely to the unfair treatment of smaller firms. Corporations, which include most large businesses, can deduct the full cost of their medical expenses from their federal and state income taxes, but these 100-percent deductions aren't available to most small businesses, which usually are sole proprietorships, partnerships or Subchapter S corporations, or to individuals.

Large companies also can negotiate effectively with health-care providers and insurance companies for lower costs for their medical programs, but these savings for big firms are merely passed on as additional expenses for smaller businesses and individuals.

The ability to adopt a self-insurance program likewise is limited to larger corporations with comfortable financial reserves. Self-insuring is usually less expensive, and because companies don't have to make up-front payments for insurance premiums, they can preserve large amounts of vital cash flow. And companies that are self-insured don't have to comply with the various state government mandates that are always expensive and sometimes ridiculous.

According to John C. Goodman, president of the National Center for Policy Analysis in Dallas, in 1970 there were only 48 laws on the books of all states mandating certain coverage in medical-insurance policies. Today there are nearly 1,000 different state laws pertaining to what companies must include in providing health care for their employees.

Goodman says that experts in the insurance industry estimate that if all the various state mandates were removed, the cost of health insurance would be reduced by more than 30 percent.

Coverage required by various states includes such things as alcoholism and drug-abuse treatment, AIDS, heart transplants and even acupuncture and in vitro fertilization. Some states have carried their demands to the extreme. California, for instance, requires that marriage counseling be included in health insurance policies, while Minnesota says company insurance plans must include hair pieces for bald people. Vermont requires pastoral counseling and Massachusetts insists that coverage includes the cost of sperm-bank deposits.

Many small companies in all sections of the country simply can't afford to offer health care to their employees due to the increasing costs and the fact they can't deduct the expenses from their income taxes. The Health Insurance Association of America reports that only 27 percent of companies with fewer than 10 employees offered health coverage as a fringe benefit in 1990, and the percentage is dropping each year.

The lack of medical insurance puts these small companies at a major disadvantage in attracting skilled employees. Many workers won't leave a firm that offers health care to go to work for one that has no medical coverage.

A 1992 Gallup poll for the Employee Benefit Research Institute showed that 75 percent of American workers regard employer-provided health insurance as "very important," and 68 percent of them rated health coverage as the most important benefit available. The poll also showed that 56 percent of American workers said they wouldn't accept a job that didn't provide health insurance. Those that are covered by a company health plan said they would need an average of $4,570 in added yearly pay to give up their medical insurance.

The advantages enjoyed by large companies don't mean big firms aren't facing the same long-range crisis as smaller firms. It merely means that small businesses will be forced to drop out of the health-care race before their big brothers.

And not all of the large companies are enjoying lower insurance costs, especially those with powerful labor unions to contend with. Unions naturally are unwilling to give up generous health-insurance benefits that were agreed upon years ago when costs were much lower. Attempts to increase employee contributions for insurance premiums or to raise the amount of deductibles and co-payments often result in disruptive strikes. Most labor walkouts today are due to disagreements over health coverage.

Many larger companies also face a problem with providing health insurance for retirees, something most smaller firms do not face.

Those especially hard hit are the country's large and older companies with staggering numbers of retired workers. Some of these companies, primarily those that have been forced to drastically reduce their size, are literally facing insolvency over the unaffordable costs of providing health care to retirees.

One example is Navistar International Corp. of Chicago, a manufacturer of medium and heavy-duty trucks. During the past dozen years, the company has had to reduce its work force from nearly 100,000 to its present 13,000 employees. It is providing generous health-care benefits to not only its 13,000 workers but 44,000 retired workers and 23,000 dependents.

Unable to work out an agreement with its unions, Navistar has appealed to a federal court to get permission to reduce some of the costs of retiree health insurance. The company told the court that of its $165 million net loss during fiscal 1991, $138 million was attributable to paying for retiree health-care benefits.

Even healthy companies are facing serious problems in providing benefits to retired workers. While many can afford the costs without fear of insolvency, the tremendous expense is making them uncompetitive with foreign companies. This is especially true with American auto makers and other large manufacturers and troubled airlines.

During the last few months of 1992, several large U.S. companies announced they will be taking harsh action regarding health benefits for retirees. Unisys Corp., the Blue Bell, Pa., computer company, revealed it plans to eliminate all retiree medical benefits within three years. McDonnell Douglas Corp, an aircraft manufacturer, announced it will provide health insurance for retirees who were salaried workers for only the next four years. Caterpillar, Inc., Peoria, Ill., said it is planning to limit retiree health benefits by refusing to pay for any increases after 1999.

A spokesman for Caterpillar, which manufactures construction equipment, told the *Wall Street Journal* that it "must do more to remain competitive and build a secure future."

A 1992 survey of 1,380 large companies by A. Foster Higgins Co. showed that 47 percent of them have either raised contributions by retirees for health coverage or plan to do so within the next two years. In addition, 40 percent of the firms are increasing deductibles or co-payments in their retiree medical plans.

The prevailing system of employer-funded health insurance is the rope that is slowly strangling American companies of all sizes. It is a system that probably never would have been started if not for a couple of very unusual circumstances.

The first occurred back in the Great Depression of the 1930s when health-care providers received nearly all of their revenues in direct payments from patients. As incomes shriveled, people did not have the funds to pay for medical services, and although many physicians accepted home-grown fruits and vegetables or a fat chicken, community hospitals barely survived.

Blue Cross, the first health insurer, came into existence in 1934 as a result of the depression, but most commercial insurance companies wisely regarded the concept of offering coverage for illnesses as a foolish venture.

Experts in the field argued that medical care was entirely too risky an area for responsible insurers, declaring it was impossible to accurately predict the demands for service when these demands were controlled by patients. Insurance against fires, accidents, thefts, etc., made sense because these risks didn't increase when people had insurance against them. Medical services, on the other hand, were certain to increase at an unknown rate when patients used insurance instead of cash to pay for them.

The concept of health insurance probably would have faded away if it had not been for President Franklin D. Roosevelt, who imposed strict wage and price controls during World War II.

Civilian employers, who desperately needed workers during the severe labor shortage caused by the war, were unable to attract employees by offering higher wages because of the Roosevelt freeze. They could, however, tempt workers to join their companies by offering them totally free fringe benefits, such as life insurance and health insurance.

The growing popularity of employer-provided health insurance forced commercial insurance companies to drop their opposition to it and to join Blue Cross and Blue Shield in offering the coverage.

By the 1950s it was common for U.S. companies to provide health insurance for their workers, and labor unions routinely insisted on this fringe benefit in their worker contracts.

It has taken more than 40 years to prove that insurance actuaries who originally opposed the theory of insuring medical care were correct. The time has come for citizens to again assume most of the responsibility of paying for their own medical services, with the federal government acting as an insurer against catastrophic losses.

U.S. companies will benefit immensely by removing the obligation of providing medical insurance for their employees, but so will their workers, who will be receiving the same quality care with no additional out-of-pocket costs than they are currently paying.

Most workers will be receiving pay increases if companies no longer have to pay for health care. Brad Robinson, president of Robinson Rubber Products Co. of New Hope, Minn., points how this will be achieved. Robinson says that 40 years ago, employees at his company received about 33 cents in wages for each dollar of revenue his firm generated. Today, his employees receive only 20 cents of each dollar of revenue. The other 13 cents is now going to health-care costs and government-imposed expenses such as workers compensation insurance.

Companies throughout the country also would be adding new employees if health-care costs were eliminated. Not only would the additional funds be used for expansion purposes, companies would change the trend of using overtime instead of adding new employees as production increases.

Because medical costs have become so expensive, most companies, especially manufacturers, today put their current workers on a regular overtime basis when productions increases, which is far less costly than hiring additional workers even considering that overtime requires higher hourly wages for the extra time worked.

Stephen R. Sleigh, deputy director of the Center for Labor Management Policy Studies at City University in New York was quoted in the *New York Times* recently as saying, "From the employer's perspective, it's easier to get people to work overtime, to pay time and a half, than to pay benefits for an extra employee."

The amount of overtime by U.S. manufacturers has been steadily increasing in recent years. The average per worker per week among manufacturers in 1980 was 2.4 hours, while today it is four hours. And as overtime jumps, the fulltime payrolls keep falling. In January 1989 there were 19.5 million workers in the manufacturing sector compared with only 18.2 million in July 1992.

There will be many other advantages for workers if companies aren't saddled with the cost of providing health insurance. Workers will once again have the freedom of moving from one job to another without the fear of losing their health insurance. They won't have to keep jobs they hate just because their company has a good health-insurance program. They won't have to turn down a new position because the worker's wife is pregnant or because someone in the family has a pre-existing illness. They won't have to turn down a job they might love, just because the new company doesn't provide health insurance. Workers will have the freedom to start their own business, knowing they will have the same health benefits as anyone else.

People on various welfare programs won't have to stay on the government-handout system just because their health insurance will be lost if they move to a job without coverage. There will be an incentive to accept a lower paid job if the generous welfare health program is no longer available.

More than 30 million Americans start a new job each year and under this new system the complicated problems of health insurance won't be a factor in changing jobs.

If the "Common-Sense Solution" is implemented as a replacement for our present health-care system, it would be a tragic mistake not to include the country's seriously flawed workers compensation insurance program—at the very least the medical-cost portion of it.

U.S. companies today are spending $62 billion on workers comp costs, nearly three times as much as the $22.3 billion spent in 1980 and nearly 13 times as much as the $4.9 billion in 1970. The 81-year-old workers comp program has outlived its usefulness. The system is being ruined by fraud, abuse and unnecessary expenses.

The cost of medical treatment for injured workers eats up about 40 percent of the total $62 billion paid out by employers, up from 33 percent in 1980. There is no good reason for the skyrocketing medical costs of treating injured workers. The average cost of treating a worker's injury in 1990 was $6,611 compared with only $1,748 in 1980. A study by the state Department of Labor and Industry in Minnesota in 1990 found that hospitals on average charged twice as much for an injury covered by workers compensation than for an identical injured not covered by the program. This could be corrected if the present workers comp system could be incorporated in the "Common-Sense Solution." Employers could pay the normal share of the worker's cost for medical treatment and the federal government would take care of the remainder.

Even if the workers comp system weren't included in the new health-care program, it is time to drastically reform the entire program.

More than half of the total workers comp costs today are drained away by administrative costs and attorney fees. And many of the claims made by workers are not truly injuries but outright fraud and abuse, and the rising costs are destroying many businesses and causing others to move from a high-cost state to one with lower rates.

A good example of how the workers comp system is failing can be found in the July 1992 issue of *Nation's Business* magazine. The article, by Roger Thompson, tells the story of Robert Boucher, owner of Astro Flight, Inc., in Marina del Rey, Calif., who fired two of his 17 workers in 1991 because they were "problem employees."

Shortly after the dismissals, both workers filed for workers comp benefits, claiming the firings caused them "debilitating stress." Because of the claims, Boucher's insurer abruptly canceled the company's coverage.

The article states: "In desperation, Boucher turned to the state's assigned-risk pool, which is required to take any business that can't purchase insurance on the open market. But admission to the pool came at a steep price—a 500 percent surcharge over his former premium of $18,000. Boucher had to come up with $108,000, a ruinous sum equal to nearly half his annual payroll. Because companies can't operate without workers comp insurance, he had no choice but to dismiss his work force and close down on Nov. 14, 1991."

Boucher's case is not unique. Almost any business leader can cite examples of unnecessary grief caused by ridiculous claims filed by workers, and most of them are upheld by liberal workers comp administrators and judges.

Take the case of Ruth Jandrucko of Miami, Fla. Back in 1986, Jandrucko, who was working for Colorcraft Corp., a photo processing company, was mugged on the job by a black man. Due to the mugging, Jandrucko is receiving workers compensation benefits because of "post-traumatic stress disorder."

In 1991 and again in 1992, a Florida compensation-claims judge ruled that she is incapable of working at her job because of her phobia about blacks, particularly "large black males." In December 1992, she was awarded $50,000 in workers compensation from her former employer's insurance company, and her attorney was awarded $450,000 for handling the case.

It would be a simple matter to include the medical-cost portion of workers comp into a new health-care program, and then it would be easier to correct the abuses in the rest of the workers comp system.

"Basic Right" Propaganda

6

Most Americans assume that access to quality health care with the payment coming from a third party is a basic right. Why is that? The answer is simple: Americans have been brainwashed!

Those who have been spewing out the "basic right" propaganda for the past several decades claim health care is a moral issue because it can become a life-or-death situation. Without proper medical care, a person can die.

How about food?

People die from starvation, too. They can become ill, or even die, if they don't eat enough of the right foods, but while we regard health care as a basic right, we regard food as a responsibility of the individual. It doesn't seem consistent, does it?

It's true that we have free food stamps for the nation's poor, but we also have public clinics and hospital emergency rooms that provide free health care for the poor. Americans should have a medical-care system similar to the one we use for food—those who can afford it will pay for their own medical care, while those who can't will receive it free.

If this country provided food for its citizens as we do medical care, our food-supply system would be a disaster. But because food is grown, collected and distributed in the U.S. via an effective free-market system, Americans spend a smaller percentage of their income and they eat better than people of any other country in the world.

Americans spend only 9.8 percent of their personal consumption expenditures on groceries, according to the U.S. Department of Agriculture. People in France, in contrast, spend 15.9 percent on food, while Italians spend 18.8 percent and the Greeks a whopping 31.3 percent.

A typical American family of four (husband, wife and two pre-school children) can have a nutritious diet for a cost of about $100 a week. The choice of quality food at groceries stores is varied and abundant and the service is excellent.

But let's assume for a moment that Americans received their groceries as they do medical care. Instead of paying $100 a week out of their pockets, the typical family receives "grocery insurance" from an employer as a fringe benefit. Through this insurance, the family can get all the food it needs.

There no longer would be any incentive to shop carefully to get the best food at the lowest cost. The family wouldn't have to spend hours every week clipping coupons from newspapers to save a dime or 25 cents from the regular cost of an item. Instead of buying hamburger at $1.79 a pound, the family would select tenderloin steak at $5 a pound, but because of the huge demand, the price of steak would soon soar to $10 or $15 a pound. Grocery stores would no longer stock inexpensive but nutritious food items, because everyone naturally would want the highest quality food available. Leftovers would be a thing of the past--why warm up something from last night's dinner when the insurance will provide groceries at no cost to the consumer?

Under this new food system, we would see total grocery costs soar from the present $400 billion a year to twice or three times that amount within a few years. There would be severe shortages of the most popular foods and long lines at the checkout counters. Regulators from insurance companies would be prowling every aisle in the supermarket, reviewing your shopping cart to make certain you weren't taking more than you need.

The food system would become one giant mess, just as our health system has become.

It's absolutely essential that Americans go back to a predominately free-market program for health care before our present system is ruined. Drastic reform is needed, but we can't look to other nations for ideas; we must be innovative and adopt a plan that is superior to any currently in use. A new system must eliminate the faults without destroying the successes of our present medical care.

In past years, Americans have benefitted greatly from tremendous medical progress, made possible primarily by hard-working, talented physicians, operating under a free-market system.

Nearly all significant advances in medical technology in the past half century have originated in the United States. That includes life-saving drugs, high-tech medical equipment, remarkable surgical procedures and the almost unbelievable progress in organ transplants.

American physicians are responsible for nearly eliminating many life-threatening diseases, such as polio, smallpox, and tuberculosis, and if they aren't handicapped by unworkable changes in our present system, it will be American doctors who will eventually find a cure for cancer, heart disease and AIDS.

Adopting the "Common-Sense Solution" would save the free-market aspects of our health-care system and convert it into a program very similar to the one we use for food. About 90 percent of Americans would pay directly for their medical care, while the other 10 percent would rely on the government to cover most or all of their costs. Today, 90 percent of Americans buy their groceries with their own money, while 10 percent receive government food stamps.

Those who feel that comparing food to medical care is not a good analogy have a strong argument, because there are vast differences, but the superiority of a free-market system over socialism in nearly all areas has been demonstrated countless times throughout the world.

The major difference between food and medical care is that the 10 percent of Americans who are using food stamps consume less than 10 percent of total grocery costs, while the 10 percent of Americans who would be covered by government health insurance under the "Common-Sense Solution" would consume more than half of total medical costs.

The fact that 90 percent of Americans have medical costs that represent less than half of total health-care expenditures is the overwhelming reason the "Common-Sense Solution" will work. It is convincing evidence that nine-out-of-ten Americans can easily afford to pay directly for their medical services.

The table on Page 111 shows how costs under the "Common-Sense Solution" will be paid. The data in the table are only estimates, but they are based on current official figures and most probably will be fairly accurate within a year or two after the system is implemented. The numbers represent costs for a full year.

As explained in Chapter Three, the new program could cut total costs almost in half through savings in administrative costs, unnecessary medical services and fraud and abuse, but to be conservative, the total expenditures in the table represent a reduction of only 36 percent from projected 1993 costs.

The table shows that one percent of Americans, or approximately 2.5 million people, will be responsible for about $120 billion, or 20 percent, of the $582.6 billion total expenses. Almost all of this cost will be covered by the federal government insurance program. The patients incurring these services will be those with the most serious illnesses, many of them in the last few weeks of their lives.

The second category, the 8 percent with annual expenses between $5,000 and $24,999, are mostly patients who will require hospital confinement. About 80 percent of their total costs of $240 billion will be covered by the government insurance plan.

The other 91 percent of Americans, who will have annual medical costs ranging from zero to $4,999, will be paying the bulk of their $222.6 billion out of their pockets. This means those 227.5 million Americans will be spending out of pocket an average of less than $1,000 each, which is a lower amount than most of them are presently paying through contributions toward insurance premiums, co-payments, deductibles, drugs, and other out-of-pocket costs.

On an overall basis, individuals will be spending considerably less under the new program than they do currently. The table on Page 85 shows that during 1993 individuals will be paying $316.8 billion directly out of pocket for their health care. Of that amount, $40.2 billion represents payments for the Medicare hospital trust fund that come from the individuals' share of Social Security taxes. Although Medicare will be abolished, the Social Security taxes probably won't be lowered.

Excluding the $40.2 billion in those taxes, this means individuals will be making $276.6 billion in direct payments during 1993 compared with only $222.6 billion under the new system, for a savings of $54 billion, or about 20 percent less than they are now paying.

During 1993, individuals will be paying $191.9 billion out of pocket for medical services and prescription drugs, but they also will be contributing $70.4 billion for medical insurance through employee contributions or individual policies, plus the $14.3 billion that Americans over 65 will be paying in monthly premiums to the federal government for Medicare coverage.

Although a few people will be spending more in an unusual year than they currently do under today's health-care system, most will see considerable savings, especially the 35 million who go through an entire year with no medical services at all.

The big savings, however, will be realized over a longer period of time.

Let's take the example of a typical family of four over a five-year span. The family, consisting of a mother, father and two pre-school children, are presently spending an average of $2,500 a year out of pocket through insurance premiums and other direct costs, or $12,500 for the five years.

It would not be unusual for this family to have four of the five years nearly free of medical costs, except for routine dental visits, eyeglasses and a few minor illnesses. Let's say their average costs for those four years were $500 annually. In the fifth year, one of the children required hospitalization for a serious illness that cost $25,000. In

COMMON-SENSE SOLUTION COSTS

MEDICAL SERVICES	NUMBER OF AMERICANS	AVERAGE AMOUNT	TOTAL AMOUNT
More than $25,000	1 percent or 2.5 million	$48,000	$120 billion
$5,000 to $24,999	8 percent or 20 million	12,000	240 billion
$2,000 to $4,999	11 percent or 27.5 million	3,500	96.3 billion
$1,000 to $1,999	15 percent or 37.5 million	1,500	56.3 billion
$500 to $999	19 percent or 47.5 million	800	38 billion
$1 to $500	32 percent or 80 million	400	32 billion
None	14 percent or 35 million	0	0
TOTALS:	**250 million**		**$582.6 billion**

their income category, the family would pay $4,000 of the $25,000 out of pocket, while government insurance would cover the remainder.

That means the family had total out-of-pocket costs of $6,000 for the five years under the "Common-Sense Solution" plan compared with $12,500 under the present system, for a net savings of $6,500.

Now, let's take the case of a healthy single woman who is 31 years old and is self-employed. She is presently buying her own health insurance coverage with a $500 deductible clause in it. Her annual premium cost is $2,000, or $10,000 for a five-year period. She goes through the five years with no major medical expenses and she spends an average of $250 a year for health care, or a total of $1,250 for the five years, which means her savings under the new system would be $8,750.

Those Americans who now have all, or most, of their insurance coverage paid by their employers would, in some years, pay more under the new system, but it is becoming extremely rare to find insurance programs that are totally funded by employers. It is almost a certainty that the days of zero costs for a worker will soon disappear.

Almost everyone will become a financial winner under the "Common-Sense Solution." Most individuals will save money. Businesses will save more than $200 billion a year. State and local governments will realize tremendous savings.

Even the federal government, which will be saddled with providing health coverage for those who qualify, will be able to fund the entire cost of health insurance for those who qualify without the need for new taxes.

The federal government's share of providing coverage under the new plan will be approximately $300 billion a year, or more than half of the total costs. As the table on Page 85 shows, the federal government will be spending $200.3 billion in 1993 medical costs. But this represents only the amount paid out of the General Fund. Another $101.7 billion of health-care costs are paid by the federal government from direct health-care taxes from businesses, individuals and state and local governments.

The $101.7 billion includes $41.5 billion from businesses through their share of Social Security taxes earmarked for the Medicare Hospital Trust Fund. Another $40.2 billion comes from individuals as their share of Medicare Social Security taxes, $14.3 billion from retired people for Medicare premiums, and $5.7 billion from state and local government employees in Medicare Social Security taxes.

That represents a total of $302 billion in current federal government health-care expenditures. When you add the $60 billion in new corporate income taxes that will be collected because companies won't have health-care costs to deduct, it means the federal government will have $362 billion—more than enough to fund the new program without any new taxes.

The major savings under the "Common-Sense Solution" will come, however, in future years, especially for the federal government. While experts contend the country's present health-care system will rise in cost by about 10 to 15 percent a year between now and the year 2000, the new plan could actually reduce total future expenditures as users of the program begin to realize the benefits of a free-market system.

Don't Look North

7

Various polls show that most Americans are satisfied with the quality of medical care available in the nation, but the vast majority is deeply dissatisfied with the system that delivers it. The concern by voters has prompted politicians at both the federal and state levels to put health-care reform at the very top of their list of priority items.

Dozens of different reforms are under consideration, ranging from a Canadian-style nationalized health-care plan to a program where every U.S. business will be required to provide medical insurance for employees directly or through a payroll tax.

There is one major difference between the "Common-Sense Solution" and all the other plans under consideration: The "Common-Sense Solution" will work. It is the only system that will lower costs dramatically, make health care available to everyone, and won't diminish the current high quality of medical services.

The main reason the other reform proposals are unworkable is that all of them overlook the simple fact that nine of every 10 Americans don't need any type of health insurance in any given year.

Why set up a complicated insurance program covering more than 250 million citizens when 90 percent can easily pay for their own medical services?

An efficient federally-operated health-care plan for the 10 percent of Americans who incur medical costs they can't afford to pay themselves will correct today's unaffordable, complex, unfair and failing system.

It makes absolutely no sense to have an insurance program that pays nearly all medical costs for practically everyone when most of the expenses can be paid directly by the patient, eliminating mountains of paperwork and putting the consumer back in charge of deciding what type of care he or she will need.

Many states in the country require all residents to carry auto insurance, but the policies cover only a small percentage of the total costs of owning an auto. The responsibility of buying a vehicle is up to the consumer. When you take your auto into a garage for an oil change and an engine tuneup, you pay the cost directly. You and the garage owner don't fill out dozens of complex forms and send them to your insurance company for payment. Third-party players don't step in to decide if the repairs were really needed and the costs justified.

Most people drive their vehicles for years without ever using their insurance coverage, just like Americans would do with health insurance under the "Common-Sense Solution." Auto insurance is designed to protect the consumer only in most unusual circumstances. It will protect you when you drive your $20,000 auto into a ditch and demolish it, but when a tire blows out, you pay the cost of replacing the tire. If auto-insurance policies were similar to today's health-care insurance, few drivers could afford to be covered.

Because so many Americans, including health-care providers, are intensely displeased with our flawed medical-insurance system, it seems certain that Congress will drastically change it within the next few years.

In a 1992 poll of Democrats in the U.S. House of Representatives by the Democratic Study Group, 70 percent agreed that "we should work to pass a comprehensive overhaul of the nation's health-care system." Only 15 percent of those responding to the poll said they would vote against a single-payer health-reform plan, similar to the system in Canada.

The congressmen obviously are aware of the feelings of the general public about what type of reform American voters prefer. An earlier poll of citizens throughout the country by the *Wall Street Journal* showed that 69 percent favor a national health-insurance plan copied from the Canadian system.

The U.S. House already has 71 co-sponsors for legislation to create a Canadian-style medical plan, and Sen. Paul Wellstone, a Democrat from Minnesota, has introduced a similar bill in the U.S. Senate.

But is a system modeled on Canada's national health plan an improvement over the current U.S. approach?

A Canadian physician, who is disillusioned with his country's system, adroitly describes it as "an excellent program until you get sick and have to use it." An American physician likens it to giving everyone in the country a free airplane ticket to Hawaii, and then providing only one airliner to fly everyone there.

The Canadian national health system, which has been in effect for more than 20 years, is a failure. If adopted by the U.S., it would be a disaster.

Designed to give all Canadians totally free medical services from birth to death, the system is far from being "free." The average Canadian pays 30 percent more in taxes than the Average U.S. taxpayer, with most of the higher taxes in Canada going to pay for health care.

If the United States adopted the Canadian plan, taxes here would soar even above those paid by Canadians. A February 1990 study by the National Center for Policy Analysis, based in Dallas, reported that a national health plan similar to Canada's would require at least $339 billion in new taxes.

The study said that if the U.S. used the payroll tax, currently funding Social Security and Medicare, to pay for a national health-insurance plan, the combined rate for employees and employers would soar from the current 15 percent to 29 percent. If the federal income tax were used to fund the new plan, the rate would climb by at least 14 percentage points, with the top rate for individuals going from 31 percent to 45 percent. If a national sales tax were used to pay for the program, it would require a sales tax on all goods and services of at least 10 percent.

The numbers used in the study are extremely conservative. They are based on the amount paid in 1989 directly for health care by U.S. businesses and individuals, adjusted for the higher income-tax revenue that would be received if businesses and individuals didn't deduct medical costs. Using 1993 health-care costs, the adjusted amount would be more than $100 billion higher than the study's $339 billion. That means, of course, any new taxes would be considerably higher than those estimated in the 1990 study.

Also, the study failed to take into consideration the cost of providing medical care for the more than 35 million Americans who now have no type of health insurance.

By the time Congress gets around to implementing a Canadian-style health program, it's almost certain that about $500 billion in new taxes would be required to fund it, or, even worse, it would result in a federal budget deficit approaching a trillion dollars a year. Either would be disastrous to the U.S. economy.

If congress opts for a Canadian plan, it most likely would place the largest tax burden on the backs of the country's businesses, because they no longer would be paying for health insurance coverage for employees, dependents and retirees. It's almost a certainty the new taxes would far exceed the $262.5 billion now being paid by U.S. businesses for health costs.

John C. Goodman, president of the National Center for Policy Analysis, the group that conducted the study of costs for a Canadian-style plan, says he can't understand why so many of the nation's chief executive officers are in favor of a national health plan.

Goodman was quoted in the *Wall Street Journal* as saying, "There's a naive view among CEOs here that they'll be able to turn their (health-care) burdens over to the federal government." But, he said, the new taxes "would be enormous." Goodman said that industries with highly paid workers, such as the auto industry, would end up paying proportionately more in taxes. "It's amazing to me," Goodman said, "that corporate executives aren't aware (that national health care) would entail huge taxes for their industries."

In contrast, the cost of operating the federal government portion of the "Common-Sense Solution" program would require no new taxes from either businesses or individuals, because the total cost of the government-insurance portion would be less, or about the same, as the amount now collected in taxes for the present government share of medical costs.

Even if the United States could afford a Canadian-style program, most Americans would vehemently oppose a system that is abused to the extent that patients with serious problems don't receive timely or proper treatment in too many instances.

Because health care is totally "free" in Canada, people there overuse the system. Canadians, many with minor ailments, visit their physicians there at twice the rate of that in the U.S. This, of course, would dramatically increase costs if government bureaucrats in Canada didn't react by placing severe limits on the amount of health care available, especially at hospitals and clinics.

Canadians, even those with severe problems, must wait long periods of time for proper treatment. The Fraser Institute of Vancouver, British Columbia, recently published the first comprehensive, scientific study of just how serious this waiting-for-treatment problem has become for Canadians.

The study reviewed 53 common medical procedures. It revealed that the average wait in Canada for coronary artery bypasses is 23.7 weeks, and 21.4 weeks for other open-heart surgery. The average wait for cataract surgery is 18.2 weeks, hysterectomy 16.3 weeks, varicose-vein surgery 36 weeks, hernia repair 24.6 weeks and hand surgery 12.4 weeks. Most common procedures, except for emergency, life-threatening treatment, involve long, miserable waits.

The Canadian system is the type where a man has to wait months for an operation, while he can take his dog to a veterinarian for surgery the same day. That's because, of course, the man doesn't have to pay for his own treatment, but he has to pay his dog's vet out of his pocket.

Many elderly patients in Canada don't have to wait for treatment; they simply don't receive any because of their advanced age. Dr. Isadore Rosenfeld, an American heart specialist and noted author of several medical books, knows firsthand the grief forced on people by the Canadian system.

Dr. Rosenfeld was born and reared in Canada and many of his relatives still live there. He told Gordon Slovut, a medical writer for the Minneapolis *Star Tribune*, of the plight of his mother several years ago in Montreal, Quebec.

Dr. Rosenfeld says of his mother, "When she was 78—she was a very bright, vigorous 78—she had some gastrointestinal bleeding. Her doctor in Montreal said he wasn't going to do any studies (to determine the source of the bleeding) because he might find a malignancy, and at her age there wasn't any use in treating the malignancy."

That meant, Dr. Rosenfeld said, that his mother would probably bleed to death very slowly if he left her in Canada. So he had her flown to New York. A surgeon there removed a cancerous tumor from her bowel. The cancer hadn't spread, and she recovered completely. She died at 91 of heart disease, Dr. Rosenfeld said.

There are numerous instances of Canadians fleeing to the United States for treatment they can't receive promptly in their own country due to the flaws in the national-health program.

Doctors, hospitals and clinics in the northern part of the United States routinely treat Canadian patients. Hospitals in Duluth, Minn., a short distance from the Ontario border, report that 22 percent of their elective surgeries are performed on Canadians. The renowned Mayo Clinic in Rochester, Minn., which has patients from all over the world, says that Canadians make up 15 percent of its elective surgeries. At the Buffalo General

Hospital in New York in 1990, half of its lithotripsies, which is a procedure that uses sound waves to smash kidney stones and gallstones, was done on Canadians. One of the most succinct descriptions of the Canadian health-care system was outlined poignantly in the September 1992 issue of *Reader's Digest* by Dr. Ian R. Munro, who is the director of the Humana Craniofacial Institute at Medical City Dallas Hospital in Texas.

Dr. Munro practiced medicine in Canada from 1971 to 1986 and is intimately familiar with the national health system there and its many faults.

In the *Reader's Digest* article, headlined "How Not to Improve Health Care," Dr. Munro writes: "Little Joel Bondy of Leamington, Ontario, was born with heart deformities that restricted the blood flow to his lungs. He needed open-heart surgery—soon—to live. The nearest equipped pediatric facility was the Hospital for Sick Children, four hours away in Toronto. But under Canada's national health-care system, commonly called medicare, that hospital had closed hundreds of beds. For the remaining stripped-down services, there was a long waiting list.

"After many delays, Joel's desperate parents notified administrators they were taking him to a hospital in the United States. Amid embarrassing news reports about the boy's plight, the Hospital for Sick Children gave him an early surgery date.

"But it was too late. Joel Bondy died four hours before surgery was to begin. He had waited nearly two months for his operation."

Dr. Munro also tells the sad story of Kent Maerz, a 22-year-old Calgary, Alberta, student who had keratoconus, a disease of the cornea. Kent needed a corneal transplant within a few months to correct his rapidly deteriorating vision. Dr. Munro points out that under Canada's system, the operation would cost Kent and his family nothing, but the wait would be two to three years. Kent paid the $5,000 cost to get the transplant performed at an eye clinic near Seattle, Wash. He said if he had a choice he wouldn't pay taxes for the Canadian health plan.

"When I needed it, it didn't do me any good," Kent was quoted in the article.

Dr. Munro explains that under the Canadian system, patients are ranked according to the severity of their problems. Critically ill patients, such as those who have suffered heart attacks or were injured seriously in an auto accident, are ranked "emergent" cases, and they are first in line. "Urgent" cases are next, while those not actually in danger are classified as "elective."

Dr. Munro says that while many "elective" cases are not in danger of dying, they are in pain. He quotes a Canadian physician who says, "They can survive on painkillers, but the quality of their lives is impaired, and some don't have many years left."

Even getting classified as an "urgent" case doesn't necessarily result in prompt treatment in Canada.

Dr. Munro tells the story of a British Columbia man: "On Saturday, August 25, 1990, a CAT scan revealed a mass in Stanley Robert's brain. If the mass was an abscess, it could kill within days.

"On Monday Robert's doctors decided he needed an urgent stereotactic biopsy to diagnose the mass. But the nearest equipped hospital, Vancouver General, had shut down 13 neurosurgery beds for the summer and could not take Roberts until the following Tuesday—eight days later. With Roberts visibly deteriorating, his desperate son pleaded to speed things up. But the hospital would not open an operating room after hours and incur overtime costs for staff. By Friday, Roberts was dead of an abscess."

Dr. Munro isn't alone in his feelings about the Canadian system or in his decision to leave the country to practice medicine in the United States. He said that in 1990 there were 8,263 Canadian doctors practicing medicine in the U.S.

Dr. Munro ends his *Reader's Digest* article by saying, "When an individual's medical expenses become crushing, most people believe their government should step in. But to nationalize all health care as Canada has done would be to toss our system out of the frying pan and into the fire. Patients must be free to make their own arrangements with their own doctors, or there is no hope for American health care."

Terence Corcoran, a columnist for the Toronto *Globe and Mail*, sums up the Canadian system even better. He writes, "You can believe that socialized medicine is the most moral system in the world if you want. But the fact is that socialized medicare will not work."

It's true that the Canadian system is a generally compassionate one, but human beings throughout the world are prone to take advantage of programs that are designed to protect everyone at no direct cost to them. And Canadians are definitely taking advantage of their "free" health care.

The wealthy and powerful and the poor and homeless are the biggest abusers of the Canadian system. Although health-care is rationed in an attempt to hold down soaring costs, government bureaucrats, politicians, wealthy business leaders and other influential people skip the waiting lines for their health care by contacting hospital administrators directly and demanding immediate attention.

Homeless drunks likewise abuse the system. It's common in many Canadian cities, especially in the winter, to have homeless people dial 911 from a pay phone and say someone is lying in the street. Then the person who made the call, lies on the ground and waits for the ambulance for a trip to a hospital emergency room where he knows he will spend the night in a warm, comfortable bed. One disgusted Canadian hospital attendant says,

"It's like a hotel. These bums are wheeled in from an ambulance and the first thing they ask is about what time we serve breakfast."

Drug dealers also take advantage of the generous medical system. They frequently go from doctor to doctor with phony illnesses in an attempt to get narcotic drugs and then resell them on the street.

Many of the country's poor commonly go to hospital emergency rooms instead of a physician's office, because they can call an ambulance for a trip to a hospital. The ambulance trip is free. A taxi ride to a doctor's office would cost them money.

Because of these common but costly abuses, regulators of the Canadian system reduce expenses by limiting care, by refusing to buy costly diagnostic machinery and by limiting funds for medical research.

As an example, the state of Tennessee with a population of 4.9 million people has more Magnetic Resonance Imager (MRI) machines to detect tumors than the entire country of Canada with 26.6 million people.

Americans who still believe the Canadian system should be adopted by the U.S. also overlook the vast differences in the population makeup of the two countries. Many of the serious problems in the U.S. that contribute heavily to medical costs here are insignificant in Canada.

For instance, the rate of AIDS in Canada is less than one-third that of the U.S. The male homicide rate in Canada is only one-fifth of the U.S. rate and the amount of violent crime is far below its neighbor to the south. The U.S. has 375,000 drug-abused babies born each year, while the problem is negligible in Canada.

Although the Canadian system is favored by many U.S. residents, the obvious problems and horrendous costs of a national health-care plan will make it difficult for Congress to implement it here. It's much more likely that politicians will compromise with a program that is commonly referred to as the "play-or-pay" plan.

This approach requires that all Americans have health insurance, either through their employer or through the government. Every U.S. business would be required to offer health insurance to its workers or to pay a new tax to fund the government program.

The result would be a continuation of present problems with the additional expense of providing coverage for the 35 million Americans who now have no insurance.

The new costs would be placed on the backs of U. S. businesses already struggling with unaffordable health-care expenses. The "play-or-pay" system would be disastrous to the millions of small companies that barely are able to stay in business in today's tight economy. Most of these small firms cannot afford to offer their employees health-care insurance, but under the new plan they will have to pay a new tax, estimated by some as 7 percent of their payroll costs.

An April 1992 report by the Republican staff of the congressional Joint Economic Committe predicted that a 7-percent tax on payrolls for the "play-or-pay" system will cause more than 710,000 workers to lose their jobs in the first year of implementation. The report said that 43 percent of these job losses will occur in small businesses that employ fewer than 20 workers.

The first-year direct costs of a "play-or-pay" program will result in an additional expenditure of at least $87.8 billion, according to the report. Most of the new cost will be paid by businesses.

Larger companies might find it less expensive to dump their present health-care plans and join the government program by paying the payroll tax, which would result in the government steeply increasing the tax rate to discourage such shifting.

Another proposal frequently mentioned as a solution to our crisis is referred to as the "private-market approach," although the name is misleading. The program would offer tax credits to individuals to encourage more people to buy their own insurance if they can't get it from their employers. It also would offer small businesses and self-employed individuals tax breaks to give them incentives to buy health insurance.

This system does not mandate coverage for everyone, and it wouldn't satisfy the large and vocal group that insists all Americans have access to health insurance. It also would require heavy new taxes to make up for the loss of revenue from the new tax credits. The system would, in effect, give the insurance industry an even bigger role in controlling the health care system, resulting in even higher administrative costs and an increase in questionable cost-control strategies already in place.

While politicians debate the various health-care reforms, many businesses and other private groups are experimenting with programs that promise to hold down soaring costs. Most of these programs are the "managed-care" type, such as Health Maintenance Organizations (HMOs). Managed-care plans have answered some of the problems, but they have failed to reduce total costs, only shifting them to others, and they have created many new problems for patients who are discovering they have fewer and fewer choices in selecting medical care.

Several state governments have started, or are exploring, programs to reform health care, but to date none has succeeded.

All of the various proposals to reform the U.S. health-care system, except the "Common-Sense Solution," have the same fundamentally contradictory objectives. They each want to expand our present "free" health-care system to millions of additional people, and, at the same time, cut total overall costs. These are impossible goals.

Managed Competition

8

Of all the various health-care reforms under consideration today, the one that is racing to the front of the pack is called "managed competition." Although this concept has been around, mostly in the background, for about a decade, the managed-competition plan gained immense prominence during the 1992 presidential election.

Managed competition combines many of the features of the managed-care plan, play or pay, and socialized medicine, but it is being touted as a free-market system.

The reason it is appealing to some free-enterprise enthusiasts is that the managed-competition plan promises to band together both companies and individuals into huge health-care purchasing networks, which then would negotiate the best possible prices from all medical providers—physicians, hospitals, clinics, etc., and even insurance companies and managed-care organizations.

Although those fortunate enough to get into the large networks might realize some cost advantages, supporters of the system ignore the fact that managed competition also would result in severe rationing of health care, a decline in the quality of medical services and further cost shifting to people not included in the network.

Managed competition also would continue, or even worsen, the endless flow of paperwork that now eats up a considerable amount of total costs.

Supporters of the system refer to receiving low prices from medical providers as the result of "negotiation," but for doctors and hospitals it would appear to be simple blackmail: "Give us an even lower price or we'll go elsewhere." It's almost certain that doctors and hospitals, rather than losing a huge supply of patients, would accept prices that would often be below their costs. This naturally would force health-care providers to cut corners, reducing the overall quality of their services.

President Bill Clinton endorsed managed competition as a system he would support, and his promise of making medical care available to everyone at an affordable cost is one of the reasons he won the election.

The nation's news media has been enthusiastic about the system. The *New York Times*, in an editorial, even declared managed competition as the obvious winner of the health-care-reform debate. *Business Week* magazine is supporting the concept. The *Wall Street Journal* says the plan is "seducing politicians and policy makers of all stripes."

Details of how managed competition would work vary with the group of supporters you consult, but the fundamental concept is that all employers in the U.S. would be required by law to provide health insurance to workers, even though it's been established that many small-to-medium size companies simply can't afford the costs. Those not included in employer groups would join other networks, with the costs paid by themselves or the federal government.

Guaranteeing medical care that is "free" in most instances to every American, because it would be paid by insurance companies or the government, would obviously increase the demand for health services, compounding the present problem of overuse of the system. Rationing would be necessary.

Sen. John Rockefeller, a West Virginia Democrat, was quoted in the *Wall Street Journal* on Nov. 2, 1992, as saying: "I think these purchasing pools are a big, big deal for the future. I see them changing the whole relationship between consumers and insurance companies, and forcing insurance companies to agree to quality, affordable deals with providers."

The key word in Sen. Rockefeller's statement is "forcing." Free enterprise is not a system of forcing the market to accept consumer demands; it is a voluntary agreement between consumers and providers based simply on supply and demand.

Managed competition also would give government bureaucrats an even larger role in health care than they currently have, adding new programs similar to the inefficient and costly Medicare and Medicaid plans.

Based on past experience, it's impractical to believe the costs of medical care can be reduced by expanding the role of government.

An excellent example of the wastes involved when the government is in charge was cited in the September 1992 issue of the *Health Letter*, a publication of the Public Citizen Health Research Group.

The *Health Letter* told about the case of an Illinois resident who wanted to obtain a nebulizer, a piece of medical equipment needed to treat his wife's asthma and bronchitis. A nebulizer converts a medication into a mist that is easily breathable. The federal government Medicare program covers most of the cost of such equipment for people 65 or over, which included the Illinois woman.

Her husband located a nebulizer that was available for rent at $59.64 a month, or it could be purchased for $160. Because his wife would need the nebulizer for a long period of time and the purchase price was no more than the cost of renting it for 80 days, the man naturally decided that buying it was the most cost effective.

He was outraged when he learned Medicare would not pay for the purchase, but it would pay for the rental for an unlimited amount of time. The supplier told the man that his store was currently renting 65 nebulizers to Medicare recipients, some of them for as long as four years.

The *Health Letter* editors investigated the incident and learned from the U.S. Health Care Financing Administration, which oversees Medicare, that it is aware of the huge waste involved in renting instead of buying such equipment, but it told the editors that the payment rules are mandated by federal law.

The editors also learned that, during 1991, Medicare paid $86.5 million just for the rental costs of nebulizers, wasting millions of dollars because of renting instead of buying the equipment.

This, of course, is just one of hundreds of examples of how government involvement adds to the total overall costs of health care.

Another recent example would be humorous if it didn't demonstrate how government bookkeeping wastes billions of dollars every year. In a letter to the editor of *American Medical News*, published Sept. 14, 1992, Dr. William I. Glass of Fairfield, Conn., wrote: "I received a statement from the Connecticut State Welfare Department, indicating that for one patient I had a credit balance of $11, and for another owed them $11, together with a check for $0. Needless to say I never deposited the check, but kept it as a treasured souvenir."

Giving government bureaucrats an even larger role in the nation's medical-care system, as promised by managed competition, would be disastrous.

The managed-competition plan evolved from a series of meetings of physicians, academics, economists and insurance executives at Jackson Hole, Wyoming, the home of Dr. Paul Ellwood, one of the originators.

The concept originally was a simple one, but it has been greatly expanded as more and more "experts" joined the group to "fine-tune" the system. It is a good analogy to the old story of a committee that was formed to design the horse but instead came up with the camel.

The latest "hump" added to the plan is a proposal by President Clinton, supported by many in Congress,to establish a national health-care board that would decide on price controls for all medical services, an idea that is strongly opposed by the originators of managed competition.

Another area of disagreement among proponents of the system is the ranking of physicians and hospitals by their patient-death rates. The original managed-competition plan was based on large networks buying medical services not only at the lowest costs but from those with the best record of quality. But how do you rank quality?

One controversial plan is already underway in Pennsylvania: a state-operated ranking system. A Pennsylvania health-data agency rates individual physicians in the state according to death rates.

The agency's first study involved 170 cardiac surgeons who performed 14,895 heart-bypass operations at 35 hospitals in Pennsylvania during 1990. The rankings list the doctors with the most deaths, those with the least deaths and those with an accepted level of patient mortality.

Physicians naturally oppose publicizing their rankings according to death rates, because there are many other factors involved besides the expertise of the individual surgeon. A doctors who is unlucky enough to have several seriously ill patients obviously won't have as good a record as one who has several relatively healthy patients. Older patient in generally bad health are less likely to survive a heart operation than a younger patient with an uncomplicated heart problem, even with the same surgeon.

If national rankings of physicians according to their patient-death rates were published on a regular basis, and the long-range success of doctors hinged on these rankings, it can be assumed that many physicians would refuse to treat a patient who had less-than-average survival expectation. This hardly is a way to improve the quality of health care.

The philosophy of managed care would play a major role in the new managed-competition plan, but it has already been proved that managed care is not an effective method of reducing medical costs.

Kathryn Langwell of the U.S. Congressional Budget Office, after a lengthy study of managed-care programs, recently stated that even if all Americans were covered by managed care, there would be little impact on total health-care costs.

In the mid-1980s, managed care was successful in cutting costs by reducing excess in-patient hospitalization, but it now appears this tactic merely shifted overall costs by greatly increasing the amount of out-patient hospital services.

Proof that managed care isn't working can be found in a new Conference Board survey that showed 69 percent of companies offering health insurance to employees now use managed care, up from 57 percent in 1989, but annual costs for those firms have been increasing at about the same rate as those of companies not using managed care.

The biggest stumbling block to managed care is its inability to control wage increases of health-care workers. Because the demand for skilled workers exceeds the supply, annual payroll costs for employees of health-care providers have been running at about double those of most other industries.

Some believe the role of managed-care organizations is cost-effective because they discourage unnecessary medical care and they refuse to pay for services that consumers should pay themselves, but there have been too many examples of failures in these areas.

For instance, *Managed Healthcare News* reported in late 1992 that "most managed-care organizations have yielded to competitive pressures and have agreed to pay" for the new nicotine patches used by people trying to quit smoking. This means, of course, that healthy individuals who want to quit smoking will have their medical insurance pay for the patch instead of paying for it out of pocket.

A 12-week supply of the patch costs as much as $300. The usual length of treatment is 12 weeks. Why should insurance pay for the patch? It certainly isn't because ex-smokers can't afford to pay for the treatment themselves. The average smoker, who has to give up his habit during the patch treatment, is saving about $360 in cigarette money in a 12-week period.

Managed-care officials defend the decision to pay for the patch by pointing to long-range health-cost savings by getting people to stop smoking. Unfortunately, studies of people who have used the nicotine patch show that only 17 percent of them are still not smoking a year after the treatment.

The original concept of managed competition, which didn't include government-mandated price controls or many of the other features being added by various groups, was a much better plan than the hybrid that has evolved. There is little chance, however, that any simple overhaul will be considered, because the most powerful groups behind managed competition are insisting on a marriage of both the good and bad aspects of the system.

One of the most influential groups supporting the hybrid managed-competition plan is the National Leadership Coalition for Health Care Reform, based in Washington, D.C. The honorary co-chairmen of the group are former presidents Jimmy Carter and Gerald Ford. The organization is also composed of several large U.S. corporations, some of the country's most powerful labor unions, the American College of Physicians and the American Association of Retired Persons.

Even though the coalition is convinced that managed competition is the ultimate answer to rising health-care costs, it admits there are serious problems involved.

In an article in the Nov. 19, 1992, issue of the *New England Journal of Medicine*, writers representing the coalition stated:

"We recognize that managed competition, promising and exciting as it is, has two limitations. The first, not a surprise, is that fundamental restructuring of the health-care system will take years to achieve. The Jackson Hole Group, which has been at the forefront of the managed-competition movement, calls its proposal 'The 21st Century American Health System,' and not without reason. The problem is not that the effort is not worth making. Clearly it is, and that is why we support it. But during the transition period, as the institutional requisites of managed competition permeate the system, costs can continue to rise unchecked in the absence of other measures to control them. At current rates of growth, they will double in six years to more than $1.5 trillion.

"The second limitation of managed competition is that it cannot work everywhere. It requires a critical mass of health-care consumers, estimated to range from 200,000 to 500,000. Without that critical mass, an area cannot support enough separate groups of 50 to 100 physicians each and enough separate hospitals to generate the competition that is at the heart of the managed-competition model."

Unfortunately Americans can't wait several years to drastically overhaul a badly deteriorating health-care system, and they don't need a substitute system that will work only in parts of the country for part of the population.

Nursing Home Care

9

The rising cost of providing long-term care for the nation's elderly and the disabled is one of the most ponderous obstacles blocking a solution to the U.S. health-care system.

In 1993, Americans will be spending approximately $73.4 billion on care for 1.9 million residents in the country's 15,324 nursing homes plus another $11.8 billion on home health care for the elderly and disabled.

The 1993 nursing-home costs are more than double those just 10 years ago, but the most frightening aspect of the problem can be found in the demographics of the nation's elderly. Today there are 32 million Americans over 65 years of age, but that number is estimated to be 60 million by the year 2030. Federal agencies have estimated that nursing-home costs will more than triple between 1990 and 2000.

If rising expenses can't be contained, the future costs of caring for the elderly will soar in a geometric progression that will make it impossible to provide the quality care needed by a population that continues to get older each year.

Although more than half of Americans in nursing homes today are 85 years or older, this also is the fastest-growing age group in the U.S. population, according to the federal Census Bureau. In the decade between 1980 and 1990, the 85-and-over population group increased 38 percent, compared with 20 percent for the 65-to-84 group and only 8 percent for those under 65. Since 1960, the number of Americans 85 and over has leaped by 232 percent, while the increase for the entire population was only 39 percent.

Back at the turn of this century, of all Americans over the age of 65, only 4 percent were older than 85. Today, more than 10 percent of the elderly are older than 85—about 3 million people. Most of the that change has taken place since 1950.

Not only are there more older people needing nursing-home care, but rules and regulations governing the payment of the costs are becoming more relaxed. Both of these elements are causing nursing-home costs to soar.

The average cost of one year in a U.S. nursing home for one person is now $38,600, a number that has been steeply climbing in each of the past two decades.

Government programs, primarily Medicaid, pay 53 percent of total nursing home costs today, while patients are paying 44 percent of the costs and insurance companies pay 3 percent.

Many nursing-home residents who have all their costs paid by Medicaid could easily afford to pay some or all of their expenses, but because of the liberal Medicaid rules and regulations, they elect to allow the nation's taxpayers to foot the bill.

Current Medicaid rules allow an elderly person to "spend down" or to protect his or her assets so they can qualify for full government benefits. The growing popularity of shifting assets to relatives so an elderly person can qualify for Medicaid is fed by the faulty conception that it's a "must" to leave an inheritance to children.

Entirely too many of the elderly say, "I want to leave the kids something, but if I go to a nursing home, they won't get anything." Then they discover they can follow government rules and go to a nursing home and still leave their children an inheritance.

The elderly can achieve the best of both worlds by "giving away" their wealth to their children before they enter a nursing home, either through gifts, an irrevocable trust and/or by purchasing an expensive home that will be inherited by the children.

By "spending down" to the amount allowed by Medicaid within the time limits required, a wealthy person can qualify for free taxpayer-funded nursing-home care.

Armond Budish, a Cleveland, Ohio, attorney and author of the book, *Avoiding the Medicaid Trap*, points out that arranging an older person's finances to evade nursing-home costs is "crazy but not immoral." He says, "If the government allows it, it can't be immoral."

Many others disagree. Stewart Bainum Jr., chief executive officer of Manor Care, Inc., a provider of long-term care, says the big fiscal threat to the nursing-home system is not the growing population of the very old, but the number of lawyers specializing in passing the burden from well-off families to the taxpayer.

Bainum was quoted in the April 7, 1992, edition of the *Wall Street Journa*l as saying: "One of the reasons costs are exploding is because it's become rather easy for upper-middle-class families with net worths between $200,000 and $600,000 to qualify for Medicaid. Bainum believes it would be wise "to bring Medicaid back to what it was envisioned to be—a safety net, and not an entitlement program."

Bainum adds: "Right now, in most states in the country, what's happening is that public-assistance funds are being used to indemnify the inheritance of the heirs of upper-middle-class parents. We see it in virtually all of the markets in which we operate. There's a cottage industry of attorneys out there specializing in this, ripping off the Medicaid funds of the states. What they're advising their clients (the parents) to do in many cases is to buy a luxurious home that's very expensive, pay off all the debt, so that they have a half-million-dollar house with no mortgage, and they can retain all that and still have $2,000, and they can qualify for Medicaid."

To obtain Medicaid benefits for nursing-home care, a person does not have to count as disqualifying assets his or her home, household goods, a car, some life insurance, and money that has been legally transferred to his or her heirs.

Partly because of these liberal rules, 35 percent of all people entering nursing homes today qualify immediately for Medicaid. Another 15 percent spend down to Medicaid eligibility within one year, and another 10 percent after the first year.

No consideration is given by Medicaid rules to the wealth of the nursing-home resident's children. Even if the person's children can easily afford to keep their parent in a nursing home, the law ignores the wealth of relatives of the patient.

Take the case of Ida, an 89-year-old widow with four grown sons. Her husband died 20 years ago and Ida has been living in the family home by herself since his death. Her only income is from Social Security. After a fall and a lengthy stay in the hospital for a broken hip, it was decided by Ida's sons that she should go into a nursing home.

Other than her home and furnishings, Ida has no assets, but all of her sons are well off financially, three of them, in fact, are millionaires. There would be no hardship for the sons to pay the full cost of her stay at the nursing home, but they, like most children, elect to have Medicaid pick up the bill.

This is legal, but is it moral? The question probably can't be answered, but the problem can be solved by changing the laws so children are financially responsible for their parents if they are reasonably able to do so.

This is not a radical suggestion. It wasn't too long ago that the culture of our society dictated that parents cared for their children when the children were young and the children cared for their parents when the parents became old. Today our culture follows a legal code instead of the old moral code.

Unfortunately, today's liberal laws, while they might win politicians a lot of votes from people of all ages, are slowly destroying the world's highest quality medical care.

Most Americans agree that the general public should pay the cost of caring for older citizens who are unable to afford to meet these expenses themselves or who have children who likewise can't afford them, but taxpayers should be spared the cost when it isn't necessary.

Under the "Common-Sense Solution," laws governing long-term care should be removed from federal supervision and shifted to states and local governments and the private sector.

The elderly who need nursing-home care or home health care should be required to pay these costs unless they can prove to local authorities they, or their families, cannot afford the expenses.

Businesses, which will have no government-imposed obligations to pay for regular health-care costs under the new system, and nonprofit organizations should play an increasingly important role in establishing quality long-term care programs at the local levels.

Corporations already are banding together to meet this challenge. It was announced in September 1992 that 109 U.S. companies had formed a partnership designed to make major improvements in the quality and availability of care for the elderly and in day-care services for children. It is the largest corporate collaboration of its kind, and it demonstrates what the business community can do in helping to solve community problems.

The corporate group, which raised $25.4 million for its program, is led by such business giants as International Business Machines (IBM), Amoco, Exxon, Sears Roebuck, American Telephone and Telegraph (AT&T), Xerox, American Express, Johnson & Johnson and Motorola.

The partnership promises to raise standards for elder-care services and to lay the groundwork for future community projects throughout the country.

If current expenses now paid for health care for employees were lifted from the backs of businesses, corporations would have billions of dollars available for voluntary programs to improve health care for the elderly and disabled and for all Americans.

If the business community could play a more important role in designing local programs for long-term care for the elderly and disabled, it's certain the programs would be more efficient than the current system.

And individuals, who would have an incentive to seek the best care available at the most reasonable cost, would turn to less costly home health care or special retirement homes instead of expensive nursing homes.

Studies have shown that only 26 percent of current nursing home residents need the costly, intensive care available there. The others could live more comfortably at far reduced costs in their own homes with professionals visiting them and taking care of their needs, or in retirement homes where minimum care is available.

Home health care already is a rapidly growing industry in the U.S. and could become the most common form of elderly care in the future. Today there are more than 5 million people already receiving home-care services. There are more than 11,000 home-health-service providers in the country, and many hospitals are beginning to offer these services.

According to the American Hospital Association, the number of hospital-run home-health-care programs has tripled in the past 10 years because of new technology, the growing number of elderly people and AIDS patients, and efforts to cut high hospital bills. The Medical Center at Princeton in New Jersey says its home visits have doubled since 1987.

It costs only about $750 a month for routine skilled nursing care at home compared to an average of $3,200 a month for nursing-home care.

Removing federal bureaucrats from regulating nursing homes would drastically reduce overall costs without lowering quality care.

J. C. Michael Jr., a Wayzata, Minn., nursing home owner points out how government interference has caused costs to soar in recent years.

Michael wrote an opinion article for a newspaper recently. He said, "I own a nursing home that has been in operation very successfully for the past 40 years. The first 20 years were relatively simple. We charged a fair rate and were paid without question by individuals or county welfare agencies. During this time we were able to pay our employees well, pay all our bills, and set money aside for alterations or improvements."

Michael adds: "Then came the Social Security Act of 1968. This bill put the federal government right in the middle of our business. The result has been a spiraling of regulations and a tremendous increase in costs. At this time our rates were less than $10 a day. We had a registered nurse as head nurse, who was on from 7 a.m. to 3 p.m. daily. Each shift had one licensed nurse in charge. Our nurses' aides were given 1.5 to 1.7 hours of aid time per patient day. The care given was constantly praised and complaints were few.

"The nursing home was under the direction of doctors, not the government. They (the doctors) saw to it that necessary records were kept, that the staff performed well, that diets were good, and that the residents were well cared for. Then came the bureaucracy. Into the U.S. Department of Health and Human Services moved thousands of social workers and attorneys. The first impact we felt was an immediate increase in record keeping.

"I asked a representative of the health department why we needed all this extra record keeping? She answered, 'Well, you want to be protected if you are sued, don't you?' We had never been sued for anything. This seemed such a waste."

Michael said that before the bureaucrats took over, his nursing home had three licensed nurses on his staff for his 100-bed nursing home. Today, he is required to have 10 licensed nurses. The additional staff devotes more of their time to record keeping than to caring for patients.

This is just one example of huge government waste in the operation of nursing homes. The government rules and regulations are strangling the industry. For instance, a recent regulation required the spending of $325 million for vaccinating all nursing home employees throughout the country to prevent hepatitis B, but there hasn't been a single documented case of patient-to-staff transmission of this disease.

Local control of nursing homes and other long-term-care operations, along with shifting more of the expense directly to individuals, will most certainly help contain the soaring costs in future years.

Eliminating Medicaid financing for long-term care will result in additional costs for those who today are evading any out-of-pocket expenses, but the horror stories of potential financial destruction for many families simply aren't true. Those who can't afford long-term care will receive public assistance, and most of those who can afford to pay directly aren't looking at years and years of expensive treatment.

A recent study showed that 30 percent of today's nursing-home residents either returned to their own homes or died within the first three months of admission, and more than half either returned home or died within the first six months.

While scaremongers want us to believe that nearly all Americans will end up in nursing homes eventually, the facts paint a very different picture. Only 2 percent of Americans between 64 and 75 currently reside in nursing homes, and only 20 percent of those 85 or older live in one. Most of the elderly never will require expensive nursing-home care.

The country definitely needs a good program that will protect families from financial ruin because of necessary care for the elderly, but those who can easily afford to pay this expense should be required to do so.

Another health problem that sometimes involves long-term care is mental illness. Under the "Common-Sense Solution," patients suffering from mental illnesses will be covered by the federal insurance program in the same manner as patients with physical problems, but the decision of who should receive in-patient care at hospital psychiatric wards or institutions for the mentally ill should be carefully monitored.

Because most psychiatric treatment is paid by insurance or public assistance, there has been a growing amount of fraud and abuse in the treatment of mental patients in recent years. The American Psychiatric Association estimates that $34 billion was spent in 1989 on hospital-based psychiatric care, with about 67 percent paid for by private insurance, 17 percent by Medicaid and Medicare, and only 16 percent paid by patients.

One study shows that between 1984 and 1989 the number of private psychiatric hospitals rose from 220 to 403, an 83-percent increase, while the number of psychiatric units in general hospitals increased from 1,259 to 1,858, a 47-percent increase. The larger number of beds has resulted in more liberal admission policies, often resulting in unnecessary treatment.

A 1992 federal government review of private psychiatric hospital cases found that in 64 percent of the cases, patients never should have been admitted, were kept longer than necessary, or the hospitals could not justify treatment with their medical records. The study also described as widespread the practice of changing diagnoses to fit insurance coverage, and the changing of a patient's diagnosis to "cured" on the day their insurance coverage ended.

Many mental patients in hospitals and other institutions could be treated just as effectively with out-patient care, and although this decision should be made by physicians and the families involved, it's obvious that thorough reviews are necessary.

Patients with mental illnesses, just as those with physical illnesses, should have quality treatment available to them at affordable costs, but unnecessary care must be eliminated whenever possible.

Other Health Services

10

In establishing a drastically reformed health-care system, most attention naturally is directed at hospitals and physicians where the largest share of today's costs is funneled. How about other areas, such as dental services, vision care, chiropractic services and treatment for alcoholics and drug addicts?

Although these peripheral services represent only about 10 percent of total health-care costs, they have become increasingly serious problems in recent years, primarily because of attempts by insurance companies and government bureaucrats to control costs.

This is especially true in dental care and chemical-dependency centers, where third-party interference has led to a wide range of problems.

The obvious solution is to exclude all four of these areas from the program governing physicians and hospitals where federal government insurance protects everyone from catastrophic costs. There seldom are such costs in dental and vision care or chiropractic services. Treatment for alcoholics and drug addicts can be expensive, but past experience of having insurance companies or government programs involved has been extremely disappointing.

Excluding these areas would result in less record-keeping, lower costs, improved treatment, and total control by the professionals and their patients who have been losing that control to third-party administrators.

There would be exceptions to this exclusion. The vision-care expenses that would be the sole responsibility of the patient are confined to obtaining eyeglasses; it doesn't include cataract surgery or other treatment of eye diseases by ophthalmologists. These costly procedures would be eligible for the government insurance program, as would certain expensive dental treatment such as braces for children and other orthodontic procedures, gum surgery, dentures and dental implants.

About $90 billion is being spent in 1993 on dental and eye care, chiropractic services and alcohol and drug-abuse programs, and only a small part of that would be covered by the government (eye diseases and costly dental procedures). That doesn't mean, however, that individuals would have to pay all of the remaining costs.

The business community, non-profit groups and schools would undoubtedly get even more involved than they currently are in programs for dental and eye care for children and in chemical-dependency programs.

It would not be surprising to see U.S. businesses play a much more active role in programs to treat alcoholics and drug addicts because of the huge savings that would result. Alcohol and drug abuse by employees is extremely costly to most U.S. companies in terms of absenteeism, accidents, lowered productivity, and higher medical claims.

The National Institute on Alcohol Abuse claims there are 7.5 million active alcoholics and another 10.2 million displaying symptoms of alcoholism in the nation's civilian labor force of 124.8 million. There also are millions of workers who routinely use illegal drugs, although there is little agreement among experts as to the exact number.

The National Center for Health Statistics estimates the economic costs of alcoholism in the U.S. are growing and will reach $150 billion by 1995, with about half of the loss due to lost employment and reduced productivity. Treating alcoholism and drug abuse is expensive, but the total amount spent in the U.S. is a small portion of the $150 billion loss. The most recent figures show that $8.7 billion is being spent annually on alcohol treatment and support; another $2.6 billion is being spent each year on drug treatment and support.

For individuals needing inpatient treatment for alcoholism or drug abuse, the cost is relatively high. A typical 28-day stay at a chemical-dependency treatment center costs between $7,000 and $10,000. Outpatient treatment is much less expensive, of course, but many experts claim it also is less effective.

Many companies are willing to cover the cost of substance-abuse treatment for their employees, but they also are becoming leery about the growing trend of placing people in expensive treatment centers with little regard to the actual needs. Because insurance often covers the cost, the number of treatment centers has been mushrooming until recently. The centers, which not only treat the addicts but also members of their families, who are labeled co-dependents, expanded vigorously during the early 1980s.

The number of beds available nationally at substance-abuse treatment centers more than doubled between 1978 and 1984, and the membership in the National Association of Addiction Treatment Providers jumped from 230 to 700 between 1980 and 1988.

As more and more large corporations included chemical dependency treatment in their employee health insurance programs during the early 1980s, the use of inpatient services soared along with costs.

A survey by Medstat Systems, Inc., of companies with 5,000 or more employees showed that admission of workers and family members to chemical-dependency treatment centers jumped from 2.42 per 1,000 employees in 1985 to 3.77 in 1988, a 55.8-percent increase. During that same period, the average length of stay at treatment centers increased by 5.1 percent and total costs jumped 129.3 percent.

The turning point came in 1989 when costs for chemical-dependency benefits soared by 47 percent for large U.S. companies and 18 percent for smaller firms.

Most companies began to cut back on alcohol-abuse costs starting in 1990 by using managed-care and utilization-review programs. Today only about 50 percent of beds in the nation's chemical-dependency treatment centers are filled, while outpatient services are growing.

The lesson to be learned is that when any health-care treatment is available at little or no cost to the individuals involved, overutilization of that treatment is a certainty.

That's why it's important that chemical-dependency services be paid by the people needing them or by their employers with carefully regulated rules. Insurance companies or government agencies should not be allowed in programs that are easily abused.

Dental care is another area where it's apparent that insurance coverage through companies or the government is not working. An increasing number of insurance plans are including dental coverage today without improving the quality of care but definitely increasing the overall cost.

The National Institute for Dental Research reports that employer-sponsored dental insurance covers nearly two-thirds of today's work force, up from only 4 percent in 1970. Total costs for dental services in the U.S. have doubled since the mid-1980s and will reach about $41.4 billion in 1993.

On a per capita basis, dental services cost $165.60 annually, but companies are paying an average of $331 a year for dental insurance for each employee.

If individuals were responsible for all dental care except the very costly procedures, it would reduce total costs without placing an unaffordable burden on U.S. families.

This system also would correct the problems being created by the government's Medicaid program, which has been cutting back on the amount it will pay for dental services to the point that most dentists refuse to accept new patients with Medicaid coverage.

Nearly all U.S. families also could easily afford the costs of obtaining eyeglasses or receiving chiropractic services. For those who can't afford dental care, eyeglasses or chiropractic care, there should be community programs at the local level sponsored by non-profit and charitable groups to meet these needs.

Having government programs or insurance coverage for health-care services that most people can easily afford to pay themselves cause far more problems than they solve.

Malpractice Reform

11

On Dec. 14, 1799, George Washington, the first president of the United States (1789-1797), awoke at his home in Mount Vernon, Va., with a severe sore throat. He could barely talk. His doctors were summoned, and they immediately diagnosed the problem as "inflammatory quinsy." (Modern-day doctors believe Washington probably had a streptococcal infection of the throat).

The three physicians attending the man who was to become known as the "Father of His Country" agreed he was seriously ill. They decided on aggressive treatment, starting with draining a cup of blood from Washington's veins. Then the doctors rinsed his throat with a mixture of vinegar and some dried dead bugs. Twice more during the day the doctors bled the ailing 67-year-old former president. They also dabbed some mercury on his inflamed throat.

By late afternoon Washington was feeling so miserable he insisted the doctors leave him alone. "Let me go quietly. I cannot last long," he said.

Shortly after 10 p.m. Washington died.

Much has changed in the field of medicine since George Washington left this world. There have been amazing improvements in the treatment of most diseases, and there also have been some declines in other areas of health care.

For instance, no one even considered suing Washington's physicians for malpractice. After all, his physicians were practicing the state-of-the-art medicine; they were diligent and conscientious in their treatment, and it was unthinkable back in those days to sue a doctor for doing his best.

Today when something goes wrong during the medical treatment of a patient, it's not uncommon for malpractice attorneys to be visiting the family shortly after the funeral director completes his duties.

It's not necessary these days for a physician to be grossly negligent in treating a patient before getting sued for malpractice. If something goes wrong, there is a good possibility someone will be sued today regardless of the circumstances.

And it isn't just physicians who are the targets of today's litigation explosion in the U.S.; hospitals, nurses, and practically everyone involved in delivering health care face the unpleasant prospect of becoming defendants in malpractice lawsuits.

To demonstrate how much things have changed since the days of George Washington, let's look at a modern case of a patient with a sore throat.

A 55-year-old patient recently went to a hospital emergency department in Texas complaining of a sore throat, difficult swallowing, a 102-degree fever and chills. A physician on duty at the hospital noted the patient was "probably septic" and had a "very tender anterior neck."

In an article about the case in the Aug. 17, 1992, edition of the *American Medical News*, it was reported that the physician immediately conducted a thorough examination and diagnosed the patient's condition as acute pharyngitis and ordered a throat culture and injections of penicillin and Bicillin.

The article reported: "The patient went into respiratory arrest five minutes after he was given the antibiotics. The emergency physician ordered epinephrine administered into the heart. He was able to visualize with a laryngoscope that the patient had a complete obstruction of the airway. He was unable to place an endotracheal tube, so he performed a tracheostomy. The incision was larger than the tracheostomy tube, which had to be held in place by a nurse. About five minutes elapsed from the time of the airway obstruction until an airway was established. The acute hypoxia caused irreversible brain damage."

The physician and the hospital were sued by the patient for malpractice. Attorneys for the patient contended that the doctor should have diagnosed epiglottitis instead of acute pharyngitis and should have intubated the patient to prevent respiratory failure. The attorneys also claim that the tracheostomy was not properly performed.

A Texas jury awarded the patient $11,150,000 in damages.

It's obvious that mistakes were made in the treatment of this patient, but it's also obvious the physician and others attending the patient weren't grossly negligent.

Mistakes occur in every occupation, but when a physician errs, millions of dollars can change hands.

There are 900 new malpractice lawsuits filed every day in the United States against medical-care providers, and the average award for those winning these suits is $300,000.

The widespread growth of malpractice lawsuits and the astronomical sums involved in settling these cases are posing a serious problem in the country's medical-care system, with very few people gaining and nearly everyone else losing.

Dr. Mark Gorney, medical director of the Doctor's Company of Napa, Calif., was quoted in a Jan. 7, 1992, letter to the editor in the *Wall Street Journal*: "Out of every malpractice dollar expended, 72 cents goes to the legal community and 28 cents winds up in the injured patient's pocket."

The costs involved in malpractice suits are enormous. Physicians today are spending more than $6 billion a year for malpractice insurance while hospitals and other institutions are spending another $2 billion. Insurance premiums have jumped by more than 300 percent since 1982. The average amount paid by self-employed physicians for malpractice insurance is now more than $16,000 a year. Doctors in high-risk areas, such as obstetricians, pay between $50,000 and $100,000 a year for their insurance.

And premium costs are only a small part of the total expenses of battling the runaway problem of suing doctors when mistakes are made. Most of the costs are a result of practicing "defensive" medicine, which today is costing Americans an unnecessary $21 billion a year.

Ted Van Dyk, a Washington, D.C., public policy consultant, defines "defensive" medicine as "the proliferation of redundant tests and procedures undertaken to protect physicians and hospitals from malpractice suits." A recent survey showed that 66 percent of U.S. physicians admit they order more diagnostic tests, 54 percent schedule more follow-up visits, and 70 percent order more consultations to protect themselves from lawsuits.

The growing trend of filing malpractice claims is not only costly, but it is morally wrong. The lawsuits often punish hard-working, well-meaning physicians for mistakes of nature, or for the lack of technology yet to come. Physicians today not only have to constantly deal with the stress from the pain, suffering and even death of their patients, they also have the additional stress of being sued if anything goes wrong, even if they aren't at fault.

A sorrowful account of a physician suffering from the dilemma of being involved in a malpractice suit was dramatically related in an article in the Sept. 7, 1992, edition of *American Medical News.* Dr. Richard E. Waltman, a Tacoma, Wash., family physician, gave this account of his woes in battling a legal claim:

"In the next few weeks, it appears I will settle a malpractice claim for a six-figure amount, although I'm convinced that I did a very good job for my patient and I sincerely believe that I'm completely innocent of the malpractice charge.

"Why was I sued?

"Because a university hospital prematurely discharged a young man who received a serious head injury in a car accident, and because they did not make good recommendations regarding his future care. (The hospital has accepted responsibility and has settled.)

"Because the nursing home that received him in transfer was simply not equipped and staffed to deal with his problems. (The nursing home also has accepted responsibility and has settled.)

"And, most of all, because I accepted the patient, feeling that in our community at that time I was the physician most likely to help him and that I had an obligation to help this nursing home with someone I knew would be a difficult patient for them. I volunteered for what I knew would be a difficult job, because I felt it was my responsibility to do so.

"I would make the same choice today.

"I am accused of not following the recommendations of the university hospital—recommendations we never received—and for not making sure that my orders in the nursing home were carried out—though I would have had to be there around-the-clock to have done that.

"I am also being accused of giving poor care because I was not paid enough. That one really hurts. I see my patients without paying any attention to their ability to pay. That this patient was on public assistance did not affect how I cared for him. In fact, due to problems with the public-aid office, I never received any payment at all for this patient. His pay status did, however, cause the university hospital to discharge him earlier than they would have had he been private pay, and it did cause him to be sent to a lower-quality nursing home. With better financial resources he would have been sent to a better nursing home or to a rehabilitation center.

"But most of all, I am being sued because he was my patient and had some problems beyond my control. Or, as the attorney hired by my insurance company said to me at our first meeting, 'You are accused of being there.' And I am being sued because that is what our legal system encourages. As the prosecuting attorney told me, off-the-record of course, 'Being sued goes along with being a doctor. That's why you buy malpractice insurance. Don't take it personally. You did a good job for the kid.' (He, by the way, gets 35 percent of any settlement and has already collected more than $250,000.)

"And what is the evidence of my malpractice?

"There is none. The experts brought in by the prosecution could make no criticism of my care. Most physicians who have reviewed the case feel my care was better than community standards. One prosecution expert praised my care as being exceptionally good. The nursing home stated in writing that I had done a wonderful job. The patient's mother stated in her deposition that I was the only physician who ever showed real concern for her son and that she didn't understand why I was being sued.

"So why might I settle?

"Because a physician who hasn't taken care of patients for more than 10 years is willing to state—for a large fee—that my care was inadequate and contributed to my patient's poor outcome. (Our system allows him to state his opinion but does not require him to support that opinion with fact.) A statement from him: 'No patient should ever get a bedsore. A bedsore alone is proof of malpractice.'

"Because a university-based pharmacist who has never practiced clinical medicine or pharmacy is willing to be critical of my care—also for a large fee. One of his most remarkable statements: 'A good physician doesn't worry about what drugs are approved or recommended for a particular condition; he uses what *he* decides is right.

"Because the plaintiff's attorney knows the system well and is using every trick in the book to distort the facts of the case and cast guilt on me. He has also threatened to request far more than my policy limits and cause my bankruptcy if I lose. 'Homeless' and 'penniless' are the words he used in his letter to me. How can I make my family take that risk?

"Because I am reluctant to close my office and give my patients up for a four-week trial to be held in a city 90 minutes away from my home and office. In more than 10 years I have never taken more than a five-day vacation. I can't afford the time—financially or professionally. Our attorney suggested I rent an apartment in the city where the trial would be held. How can I stay away from my family for that long?

"And because the constant flow of phone calls, letters, depositions and legal actions has taken me away from my practice and from my family. Moreover, the stress of the process is giving me headaches, heartburn and sleepless nights. I am doing less well for my family and for my patients, and I simply can't allow that.

"I am a father of two sons, and I feel very bad for my patient and his family. I cried the first night I saw him. He is a young man with many years of sadness ahead of him. But nothing I did contributed to his troubles. Indeed, by treating him as well as I did and by getting him into a rehabilitation center—where I believe he should have gone in the first place—I helped him. He is actually doing better now, and I honestly believe that part of his recovery is due to the care I gave him. I am absolutely convinced I did the very best I could for him. And given the circumstances, I don't think any physician could have done better.

"So how do I feel about settling my first malpractice case in more than 10 years of practice?

"I still have a tremendous marriage, two great kids and many wonderful patients. I have had a challenging and rewarding life. I am healthy. The sun will still come up tomorrow morning.

"But I feel terrible. I feel abused, violated and betrayed. I am tired, but I can't sleep. I am angry. I am afraid. I am very sad. For the first time in my career, I am starting to see every patient as a potential lawsuit. Right now I feel like hanging up my stethoscope, closing my office and opening up a fast-food franchise.

"I hope I change my mind. I love the practice of medicine. I'm a good doctor, and I would really miss my patients."

Dr. Waltman's feelings aren't unusual. Most doctors feel angry and betrayed after being slapped with a malpractice lawsuit when they honestly feel they were not negligent in treating their patients.

The stress of facing lawsuits is responsible for many unfortunate changes in the practice of medicine. Large numbers of physicians are taking early retirement to escape this stress, and those who remain are making changes in the way they conduct their practice, such as avoiding certain types of patients who are more likely to sue their doctors. There no longer is that trusting relationship between physicians and their patients, and for many doctors the thrill and joy of practicing medicine is missing.

Changes are especially dramatic in certain areas of medicine where malpractice suits are the most common, notably in obstetrics where lawsuits are frequently filed when a baby is born but is abnormal.

The American Medical Association reported that 63 percent of family practitioners dropped obstetric services between 1982 and 1988 because of rising malpractice-insurance costs. The AMA also reported that during that six-year period, 45 percent of general practitioners and even 36 percent of obstetricians and gynecologists stopped delivering babies because of malpractice problems.

Changes in the practice of medicine because of the legal community's involvement in the profession is becoming a hardship on all Americans by making quality medical care more difficult to obtain and much more expensive.

Are there instances where an incompetent physician deserves to be punished for grossly negligent behavior? Yes, of course, but these cases are rare, and legal action should be reserved for these unusual incidents and should not be used every time something goes wrong while a physician is doing his best.

Excessive legal action in the U.S. isn't limited to the medical field; it's rampant in nearly all areas. There were 18 million civil lawsuits filed in U.S. courts during 1991, costing the nation's economy a staggering $117 billion a year through legal fees, jury verdicts, settlements and liability insurance.

Million-dollar-plus settlements are becoming more common each year. One of the largest awards came in October 1992 when a 10-year-old District of Columbia boy won a $15-million claim after falling off playground equipment. The boy, Tyrone Ferguson, suffered head injuries when he landed on the asphalt surface. He was in a coma for a week and has recovered, but he suffers from "hyperactivity and an impaired ability to resist impulsive actions."

Attorneys for Tyrone claim the playground surface should not have been asphalt; it should be wood chips, sand or rubber matter.

The settlement calls for an immediate payment of $302,000 plus $125,000 for medical expenses. He will receive payments of $40,000 a year until he is 21. After that he will receive

$216,708 a year for the remainder of his life. On top of that, Tyrone is to receive a lump sum payment of $4.3 million.

Accounts of unusually high settlements are becoming more and more common throughout the country, especially when the lawsuits involve serious injuries or illnesses, and where medical-care providers are accused of making mistakes.

Most Americans, except those in the legal community, believe severe restrictions should be placed on the amounts awarded in malpractice suits. A survey of corporate-benefit managers throughout the country showed that 90 percent of them are in favor of revamping medical-malpractice laws.

There is little debate that when there is gross negligence involved, the patient should receive compensation for past and future medical expenses and for the loss of future earnings. But most people feel there should be limits on the amounts awarded for pain and suffering and punitive damages.

Some states already have a $250,000 limit for pain and suffering and punitive damages, but a nationwide law is needed. Other restrictions should be included in laws regulating medical-malpractice suits. Suits should be limited to those where it can be proved that "gross negligence" was involved and should not include those where innocent mistakes were made. Contingency fees for attorneys should be abolished. People who file lawsuits and lose should be required to pay the legal costs for the defendants. There should be no up-front, lump-sum payment, except for medical expenses.

If medical-malpractice reform can be enacted, the big winners won't be physicians and other health-care providers. The big winners will be all American consumers, who today are losing out in affordable and quality medical care.

Victims Not Villains

12

Despite a convincing campaign by the news media, the villains in this country's medical-cost crisis are not the doctors, hospitals, drug companies and other health-care providers. Instead, they are the victims of a system that has gone awry.

It's true there have been legitimate complaints against the people responsible for delivering health care, especially in the amounts charged for certain services, but in most instances these are the reactions of desperate people trapped in an unfair, ineffective system and not because of any moral decay on the part of the vast majority of medical professionals.

In the past, a physician's only allegiance was to the patient. Today, a doctor must not only care for the patient, he or she must satisfy state and federal bureaucrats, insurance companies, utilization reviewers, and many other third parties.

John T. Kelly, director of the American Medical Association's office of quality assurance, says physicians are losing patience with these "Big Brothers." Kelly was quoted in the *Wall Street Journal* as saying, "One physician might have to deal with 10 to 20 different review organizations a day, each of which has unique criteria for evaluating medical claims."

Dr. Robert J. Becker, chairman of HealthCare Compare Corp., a health-cost management firm, admitted in the same *Journal* article that "there's a degree of legitimacy to doctors' complaints."

In their attempts to control rising health-care costs, the ever-growing hordes of third-party players have failed, and in the process they have managed to turn physicians and other medical professionals into a steaming group of disgruntled, upset and highly dissatisfied rebels.

A wise man once said, "There are three professionals I fervently hope are happy in their work, well paid and pleased with their jobs—the surgeon who is performing my heart-bypass operation, the airline pilot who is flying my commercial jet, and the teacher who is teaching my child."

All consumers benefit when health-care providers, especially physicians, are satisfied with their working conditions and compensation.

Physicians are the key to quality medical care and to controlling overall costs. Although direct payments to physicians represent only a small part of total health-care costs, they are responsible for about 75 percent of all expenditures, because they make the decisions of who goes to the hospital, who gets the drugs and medical equipment, who receives expensive laboratory tests, etc.

Because physicians are the most visible participants, they often are the first to be blamed for the various flaws in a system they have generally opposed since the mid-1960s when the federal government first entered it in a major move with adoption of Medicare and Medicaid programs.

As costs have skyrocketed, the news media, consumers, government bureaucrats, insurance companies and other third-party players have been seeking a scapegoat. They found one in the nation's physicians. Many doctors feel the public has been conned into believing that "health care is far too important to be left to the physicians."

Much of the criticism focused on doctors has involved their compensation, which is often termed excessive and responsible for much of the rising costs. Headlines frequently charge that physicians are overpaid, that they manipulate billing procedures, that they order unnecessary laboratory tests, and that they own the facilities to which they refer their patients.

Charges that physicians are paid too much usually overlook many important facts that indicate this isn't true. For instance, total charges by U.S. physicians in 1993 will represent only 18.6 percent of all health-care expenditures. This compares to 25 percent in 1945 and 27 percent in 1929.

The average pretax income of U.S. physicians after their overhead is paid is about $164,000 a year, which is misleading because of the much higher compensation received by surgeons and other specialists. The average pretax income of physicians in family practice in 1991 was $105,645.

While total health-care expenditures during the past two decades have soared most years by 10 percent or more over the previous year and have often been two to three times the rate of inflation, this isn't true with doctors' compensation.

A recent study shows that physicians' compensation has increased at an annual compound growth rate of only 3 percent a year in inflation-adjusted dollars during the past 10 years. The Medical Group Management Association, which conducts an annual survey on physician compensation, reported that median pay increases for most primary care doctors fell in 1991 behind the rate of inflation.

Most Americans feel physicians are well paid, and even most doctors agree, but hard-working physicians object to charges they are over-compensated, especially when other highly skilled workers, such as chief executive officers of companies, professional athletes and entertainers often receive 10 to 100 times the amount paid to doctors.

The income of physicians is not a major factor in the deterioration of the U.S. health-care system, and it is not an important issue among most doctors in their outrage over the changes in their profession.

One of the main concerns of physicians today is the wasteful paperwork they are forced to do to comply with the futile attempts by third parties to control overall costs. A survey of doctors over 55 years of age showed that most of them devote about 25 percent of their time to paperwork, which is about 10 times the amount they spent filling out forms when they first started practicing medicine.

Among the most burdensome medical-review requirements facing physicians, according to the American Medical Association, are profiling of an individual physician's treatment patterns, preadmission reviews, retrospective reviews, medical-necessity reviews and concurrent reviews.

Physicians also are disturbed over attempts by various groups to control rising costs with unworkable price controls. Medicaid, Medicare and insurance companies all dictate to physicians what they can charge for various types of care, meaning that doctors are forced to charge more for services to patients not protected by the "Big Brothers."

The latest assault on physicians is the new Resource-Based Relative Value Scale, which caps the fees of physicians by the U.S. Health Care Financing Administration. This new effort is not only a method of price controls but is aimed at encouraging more doctors to be primary-care physicians (family practice, pediatrics and internal medicine) instead of specialists.

Because specialists charge more than primary-care doctors, there is the false belief that changing the mix within the profession is a sensible approach. There is, in fact, no evidence that reducing the number of specialists will improve the quality of medical care or reduce total expenditures. Primary-care physicians are a vital element in health care, but the main reason the United States leads all countries in the quality of medical care is because of the specialists. Many of the astounding advances in recent years in medical treatment and in the sophisticated diagnostic equipment used today are because of specialists.

This high-quality medical care is being threatened, however, by the increasing interference from third parties, many of them unqualified to second guess skilled physicians. It's understandable why many physicians are irate over the need for approval by outsiders before they can treat their patients. Scrutiny by outside review companies is designed to make medical-treatment decisions more scientific, but the practice of medicine is still more of an art than a science. A decision by a doctor, with the approval of the patient, is still the most effective way to treat somebody. Approval of the treatment by an inexperienced reviewer often results in delays, higher costs and, in many cases, the wrong decision.

There are now more than 300 companies offering utilization review services to insurance companies, corporations and the government, and they lack uniformity in the permission granted to doctors and hospitals.

One physician was quoted recently about reviewers in a *Business Week* article as saying, "You have poorly trained personnel who are not medically literate making decisions about people with complicated illnesses."

As outside interference and more stringent price controls grow, many physicians are thinking of leaving the profession or taking early retirement. Some already have left the field.

Dr. Thomas H. Coleman, a Denver physician, explained his decision to leave the medical profession in a distressing letter-to-the-editor recently. He wrote:

"Last December, after 41 years, I closed my private practice of internal medicine, giving my 475 active patients over to the care of several other doctors of their choice. I did not really want to do this. I am in excellent health, I keep up with the medical journals, I had a fine secretary, and I like my patients. They still call me as friends. I worry about some of them, and call to inquire how they are. They all ask me why I left.

"I answer that it was time to explore some new ambitions. But there were other reasons. Most people don't realize that the 1984 freeze of Medicare fees is still in effect eight years later. Pathetic 'increases' have never matched inflation, let alone the rising expenses of a medical office.

"In the past 13 months, Congress and the President have cooked up two budgets that arbitrarily slashed doctors' allowable charges for Medicare patients by devastating percentages. Congress then voted itself a 29-percent raise. Additional reductions are being proposed. Sixty-five percent of my income came from patients under Medicare. How would I have kept up with the increases in my office rent, my secretary's salary, my liability-insurance premium and outside personal obligations? How would I have paid for more help in the office to deal with an entirely new set of complex 1992 service codes, besides the daily harassment from Medicare's brainless rules and computerized letters?

"For Americans over age 65, Medicare is destroying the quality of care by discounting its value and distracting their doctors from patient care. A way must be devised to control not only the costs of medical services but also the wasteful costs of running a government insurance plan. It should cover the uncovered. It should not pretend to insure, at great expense, hundreds of thousands of people who can afford private insurance. Its computer programs must not be loaded with suspicion and threats for doctors.

"By what kind of preemptive law does Medicare prohibit a doctor and his patient from a mutual agreement to exclude themselves from the Medicare program and to continue an independent professional and confidential relationship for an acceptable price based on time and skill? Some of my former patients are asking me. I haven't heard a rational answer. It would save Medicare a lot of money.

"I've arranged my escape from Medicare. My former patients would like to arrange theirs. Some doctors are refusing to take them on because they have Medicare 'insurance.' I can understand why."

The Medicare mess is only one of several reasons many physicians are fed up with today's health-care system. The Medicaid system, designed to financially assist poor Americans, is in even worse shape than Medicare. Most private insurance programs are being converted to "managed-care" systems, which is nothing more than a desperate attempt to artificially place price controls on all medical services.

The "Common-Sense Solution" will put physicians and their patients back in control of the country's medical-care system, and it will eliminate entirely the aggravation and soaring costs of dealing with third parties in 90 percent of health-care cases.

Greedy or Desperate?

13

Physicians are being unfairly blamed for the woes of the country's health-care system, but, relatively speaking, they are regarded as virtual saints compared to the "greedy and arrogant" hospitals.

Doctors still have some fans defending them as hard-working, caring individuals, but there is little support remaining for the nation's hospitals. Vicious attacks by the news media, bureaucrats, the insurance industry and other third-party regulators have convinced the public that much of the blame for skyrocketing medical-care costs belongs to profit-hungry hospital administrators.

Hospitals are responsible for nearly 40 percent of total health-care costs, so it's natural much attention is being devoted to their role in a system that is rapidly crumbling.

Much of the criticism of hospitals is blatantly unfair and even inaccurate, but someone must take the blame for soaring costs. Hospitals, along with physicians and drug companies, are easier for a brainwashed public to blame than behind-the-scenes regulators.

The news media regularly criticize hospitals and their role in driving up health-care costs. Even prestigious authors have leaped on the backs of hospitals in best-selling books, notably the Pulitzer Prize winner, Walt Bogdanich, who devoted more than 300 pages to a vicious attack on the industry. His book, *The Great White Lie—How America's Hospitals Betray Our Trust and Endanger Our Lives*, is described as "a chilling exposure on how too many doctors and hospitals are more interested in making money—at any cost—than in providing the best, safest medical care."

On the back of the book's dust jacket are listed several complaints about the hospital industry, including "How government investigators came to suspect that hospitals were manipulating an arcane patient coding system to cheat Medicare out of billions of dollars," and "How federal health officials built their revolutionary cost controls on data bloated through cheating and bureaucratic bungling, producing some of the biggest hospital profits ever."

National television frequently gets into the act, too. A *Prime Time Live* news show on ABC devoted much of the program to criticizing the Humana hospital chain for its pricing policies. The program pointed out that many items provided to hospital patients had been marked up drastically.

Even Congress has been attacking hospitals for their pricing policies. Rep. John D. Dingell (D-Mich.) charged in a 1991 congressional hearing that "the now-famous $640 Pentagon toilet seat pales in the face of some of these hospital charges."

The real truth is that while hospitals might be a vehicle for driving up health-care costs, hospital administrators are not driving that vehicle. They are helpless passengers. Third-party regulators, in their attempts to hold down costs, are responsible for most of the problems in the hospital industry. Because of the regulators' constant bungling, every time they attempt to solve a problem, they create three or four new ones.

There's little argument that hospital costs are too high, but the reason isn't the desire for huge profits. Most hospitals, in fact, are non-profit organizations, and even the private, for-profit companies are struggling to survive. If hospitals were allowed to itemize their billings in a realistic manner instead of being forced to fake their charges, a typical statement would contain only these items:

Patient care — $660

Bookkeeping, administration and other unnecessary charges — $2,340

TOTAL: $3,000

A 1992 study by E. C. Murphy Ltd. of Amherst, N.Y., showed that on average, U.S. hospitals spend $78 out of each $100 of revenues on clerical, communications and administrative costs (most of that eaten up by payroll expenses) and only $22 on actual patient care. During the study, 37,474 employees at 59 hospitals were asked to analyze their jobs. It showed that 60 percent of their wasted time was caused by unnecessary paperwork and poor communications between departments. Another 20 percent was due to inefficient operating methods. Most of this waste isn't due to inefficient hospital administration; it is forced on them by the ever-increasing rules and regulations from government bureaucrats and other third-party players.

While the public perceives hospitals as greedy and profit-hungry, the facts, which are not being adequately publicized, show that the country's hospital industry is in serious financial trouble with even worse years ahead.

In a report by the Council of Hospital Corporations entitled "Why Hospitals Need Profit Margins," it is argued that hospitals require a minimum profit margin of 4 percent annually to maintain financial health and to meet their needs. This includes non-profit and community hospitals as well as for-profit hospitals. The report states that without at least a profit of 4 percent of total revenues, hospitals are unable to reinvest in personnel, equipment and technology, and they are in danger of losing their ability to adequately treat patients.

Very few hospitals anywhere in the country had profits in 1992 of 4 percent or more; many lost money. Of the 6,700 U.S. hospitals, 90 percent are non-profit or "public" hospitals and only 10 percent are operated by standard for-profit corporations. The for-profit hospitals generally outperform the other hospitals financially, but even these are having serious trouble staying out of the red.

The 1992 U.S. Industrial Outlook, a publication of the U.S. Department of Commerce, states that profit margins for the nation's for-profit hospitals dropped from 7.3 percent in 1984 to 3.5 percent in 1988. Since then, margins have barely changed, reaching a peak of 3.9 percent in 1991.

With inadequate profit margins, what happens to the ability of a hospital to care for its patients? Vic Ellison, public affairs vice president of an association of 25 hospitals in the Minneapolis-St. Paul metropolitan area, points out the consequences with a hypothetical example of a hospital with less than a 4-percent annual profit margin.

In an article in the *Minnesota Journal* newsletter, Ellison writes:

"The best way to explain the need for sufficient profit is to outline a 'what-if' scenario: What if a hospital over a period of five or more years fails to meet its minimum financial targets? Let's consider the situation of 'Acme Hospital.'

"Acme is a 380-bed hospital in a middle-class section of Metro City. Its patient-payment base is 45 percent public (Medicare and Medicaid), 40 percent private (dominated by four major health-insurance plans), and 15 percent self-pay (of which one-third is indigent care and uncollectible).

"Annual patient revenues this year will be $237 million, up from $225 million the previous year. Expenses have equaled patient revenues each of the last three years, giving Acme little financial flexibility. What problems does this create?

"There is a shortage of qualified registered nurses and licensed practical nurses. Because Acme doesn't have the money to match the 8-percent pay raises that hospitals in other parts of the country are giving their nurses, the shortage will worsen.

"Radiologists on staff at Acme request that the hospital modernize its cancer center by purchasing a dual-energy linear accelerator, the latest technology for treating cancerous tumors. The multi-million-dollar piece of equipment isn't in the budget, so the board of directors turns it down. Patients needing such specialized care will have to travel 200 miles to the nearest accelerator.

"Acme desperately needs to rebuild the 'old wing' at the hospital, which is used for mental-health services and chemical-dependency treatment, two of the hospital's most lucrative programs. It goes into the bond market for building capital, but because the hospital's financial performance is below standard, it must pay a higher interest rate, making it even more difficult to make ends meet.

"For years, the Ladies' Auxiliary at Acme has sponsored an annual fund drive to help pay prenatal and perinatal medical bills for uninsured pregnant women and their newborns. This year, the auxiliary decides to dedicate the $150,000 it raises to replace a leaky roof in the day-surgery unit—an expense that would normally be absorbed by the general operating budget.

"As you can see, lack of available resources can lead directly to an inability for hospitals to reinvest in personnel, technology, equipment, infrastructure and community services. A comparable situation would be that of a farmer feeding his seed corn to his hogs rather than planting it in the field, accomplishing short-term gain by long-term loss.

"Some people might argue that Acme Hospital should be allowed to die, believing that more efficient and effective hospitals will rise up to take its place. That argument might be persuasive, except for one fact: Acme isn't the exception, it's the rule. For every financially healthy hospital, there are several Acmes. In fact, in the Twin Cities in 1989, only eight of the 22 acute-care hospitals reached that 4-percent threshold. Eight of the remaining 14 hospitals had positive margins of less than 4 percent, while the other six actually lost money."

The bleak situation for Twin Cities hospitals pointed out by Ellison pertains to the relatively financially healthy metropolitan hospitals. Rural hospitals in Minnesota, and throughout the country, are doing even worse. In 1991, there were seven rural hospitals in Minnesota that were forced to shut down, compared with an average of one a year during the 1980s. Of the 155 hospitals in the state, 61 had operating losses in 1991 compared with 59 the year before, according to the Minnesota Hospital Association.

Conditions are as bad or even worse in most other states. Texas led the nation in 1991 for the number of hospitals that went out of business, but many states are reporting serious financial problems for their hospitals.

The Iowa Hospital Association claims many of its rural hospitals will not survive to the end of this decade. A report by the association shows that 32 Iowa hospitals operated in the red during 1991, a 33-percent increase over the previous year. The report states that three-fourths of Iowa's 81 rural hospitals lost money during 1991. The report also shows there was a 17-percent increase in the amount of bad-debt and charity cases in 1991 by Iowa hospitals. Most other states have similar problems with their hospitals.

You might wonder how it is possible for a hospital that charges $4 for a couple of aspirins that cost only pennies could lose money or earn only marginal profits. There are many reasons, but the main culprit is the federal government and its attempt to reduce overall costs by limiting payments for Medicare and Medicaid patients.

The trouble began in 1983 when the federal government decided to change the method of reimbursement for Medicare patients with the adoption of the "Prospective Payment System." Instead of paying hospitals for whatever bills the Medicare patients ran up, the new system began reimbursing hospitals a flat amount regardless of how long—or short—their time in the hospital. Other strict limitations have been placed on hospitals who treat Medicare and Medicaid patients. The new policies have drastically changed who determines the price, how the price will be calculated, and what services will be paid for. The federal government makes the decisions and hospitals are forced to comply.

Each year since 1983, hospital costs have increased but federal reimbursements have fallen behind. In October 1992, the American Hospital Association revealed that seven of every 10 U.S. hospitals will lose money caring for Medicare patients during 1993 compared with 51.7 percent in 1988. In 1986, only one-third of the nation's hospitals were losing money on Medicare.

The problem threatens to become even worse after 1993 when even deeper cuts for Medicare and Medicaid are implemented and the number of charity cases increases, with more and more Americans losing their private health insurance.

Many physicians, confronted with federal reimbursements that are less than their costs, can solve the problem by refusing to accept Medicare and Medicaid patients, but most hospitals are unable to refuse care, because they had earlier accepted federal financing for new construction, expansion or modernization.

Artificial price controls implemented by the government and private regulators are pushing hospitals to the point where many of them are treating 40 to 50 percent of their patients for less than the hospitals' actual cost.

A study by Lewis-ICF, a consulting firm, found that the nation's hospitals lost almost $35 billion in 1992 by treating Medicare, Medicaid and charity patients, and they were forced to charge higher rates to privately insured patients to cover these losses through "cost-shifting."

The study showed that hospital costs in 1992 for treating patients covered by government programs would reach $137.7 billion, but government payments would be only $115 billion. The study also found that hospitals would lose $11.9 billion on free care to the poor and others who failed to pay their bills. This loss of $34.6 billion was shifted to other patients.

The study also discovered that underpayments for Medicare and Medicaid are now twice as high as losses on free care, while a few years ago they were about the same amount.

The study concluded that this is forcing hospitals to serve as "quasi-government bodies, imposing taxes on one set of patients to cover the unreimbursed costs of another."

While all hospitals are suffering under these unrealistic price controls, rural hospitals are being hit especially hard, because federal reimbursements are less for rural hospitals than urban hospitals.

The plight of rural hospitals was pointed out to a special congressional task force in January 1992. Rep. James Oberstar (D-Minn.) and Rep. Amory Houghton (R-N.Y.) heard a spokesman for rural hospitals say, "Federal reimbursement policies are killing off rural health care." The congressmen were told that most rural hospitals serve larger numbers of Medicare patients and poor people than most city hospitals."

Rural hospital spokesmen told the congressmen it was essential that Medicare and Medicaid reimbursements be increased and that Congress reform the myriad of rules and regulations that bog down small hospitals.

Michael E. Walke, administrator of Lake View Memorial Hospital in Two Harbors, Minn., told the congressmen, "We are being buried in paper and nitpicking bureaucrats. A couple of years ago the government inspection team that visited our hospital had more members on it than we had patients in the hospital."

All U.S. hospitals are facing serious financial problems today, but the next few years are expected to reach a crisis stage for the simple reason that the "easy" cost-cutting measures have already been taken and there is little room left to further reduce expenses.

When federal government limits on Medicare payments were first implemented, hospitals reacted quickly by reducing the average length of stay for many of their patients. Between 1983 and 1988, the total number of inpatient-hospital days for all U.S. hospitals dropped by a staggering 28 percent. The reduction was greatest in 1984 and 1985, and it then began to taper off until disappearing by 1990.

The number of inpatient admissions also dropped 10 percent during the 1980s, but these reductions also have ended. Because of shorter hospital stays and fewer inpatient admissions, it was necessary to eliminate surplus hospital beds. Between 1983 and 1989, hospitals closed down more than 70,000 beds, or about 7.3 percent of total capacity, according to the American Hospital Association.

These reductions resulted in cost savings, but they were offset to a large degree by significant increases in outpatient services at the nation's hospitals. In many hospitals, the number of outpatient visits doubled during the 1980s while inpatient services declined.

Without drastic changes in the rules and regulations imposed on hospitals, there is little prospect that the quality of care can be maintained and that financial problems can be controlled.

Under the "Common-Sense Solution," with no Medicare, Medicaid or insurance programs, hospitals could regain control of their operations and could adopt a fair system of billing that would treat all patients the same and would provide enough operating profit to ensure that American hospitals will remain the best in the world.

Leave Drug Industry Alone

14

Proponents of the free-enterprise system frequently point to the U.S. pharmaceutical industry as proof that the system works admirably, and that the practices employed by drug manufacturers should be adopted by other industries.

The tremendous successes of the prescription-drug industry have set examples for businesses throughout the free world for the past half-century. Most companies in the industry are profitable; they devote as much as 16 percent of their total revenues to important research and development projects; they can afford to offer well-paid jobs to nearly 200,000 American workers, and they contribute generous amounts to charity, especially through free prescription drugs to the poor.

Because of efficient management and a philosophy of long-range planning, prescription-drug companies have been highly profitable in the past couple of decades, chalking up net-profit margins double those of firms in most other U.S. industries.

Beneficiaries of this success are not only the drug companies and their stockholders but consumers in the U.S. and most other nations. More than half of the prescription drugs used today throughout the world were developed by U.S. drug manufacturers, and they are No. 1 in the global marketplace. Much of the vast improvements in medical care today are due to the efforts of U.S. drug companies. They have even played a vital role in the unbelievable 30-year increase in average age expectation since the turn of the century. Drugs and vaccines have conquered or controlled hundreds of serious diseases since the end of World War II, saving a countless number of lives and helping people avoid lengthy and costly hospital stays and surgeries.

The impressive success of the industry, however, has resulted in a great deal of resentment, anger and disgust by many liberal politicians, government bureaucrats and private health-care regulators. With U.S. health-care costs soaring, these people want Americans to believe that drug companies are to blame for much of the rising expenses and other problems in the medical system.

The facts don't substantiate this claim. Less than 7 percent of today's health-care costs are spent on prescription drugs compared with nearly 9 percent in 1966.

The U.S. Department of Commerce, in its *1992 Industrial Outlook*, states: "Prescription-drug costs in the U.S. continue to remain a much smaller percentage of total health-care costs than in other industrial countries. While spending on health care has been increasing rapidly as a percentage of Gross National Product, spending on prescription drugs in the U.S. has remained substantially under 1 percent of GNP, just as it has for the past 25 years."

While it's true that prescription-drug prices have increased in recent years, the amount has been greatly overstated by government agencies (10.4 percent a year between 1980 and 1990, according to the U.S. Health Care Financing Administration). A review of government data by the National Bureau of Economic Research showed that the actual price increase was only 5.7 percent a year. The review's conclusion was based on the fact that government figures included only existing drugs and not new products or generic drugs, which normally rise at much slower rates.

But regardless of the amount of price increases, the cost of using a drug to treat an illness is far less than other procedures.

Jeffrey Trewhitt, a spokesman for the Pharmaceutical Manufacturers Association, was quoted in the Sept. 28, 1992, edition of *American Medical News* as saying: "Prescription drugs are the most cost-effective form of medical care. Medicines help patients avoid long hospital visits, debilitating and expensive surgeries and costly nursing home confinement."

For instance, a patient who decides to use drug therapy to treat a heart problem will spend only about $500 a year on medicine, while coronary bypass surgery costs more than $40,000. The cost of treating ulcers with medicine is less than $1,000 a year, while ulcer surgery costs about $24,000.

Opponents of the prescription-drug industry, however, refuse to accept the obvious benefits from a successful free-market system; they won't be satisfied until they can see drug manufacturers overregulated to the point where the industry will be in the same league as U.S. auto manufacturers, airlines, the savings and loan industry and television manufacturers (if there are any remaining in this country).

Leading the vicious attack on the U.S. drug industry is Sen. David Pryor, an Arkansas Democrat, who is the chairman of the U.S. Senate Special Committee on Aging. Sen. Pryor and others in his camp have successfully convinced many consumers into joining the assault on drug manufacturers with emotional, but inaccurate, outbursts. It's been easy to persuade consumers to join the battle, because they are currently paying out of pocket nearly three-fourths of all drug costs. Most other medical costs are paid by insurance companies or government programs, so consumers don't directly feel the impact from those.

Sen. Pryor has been widely quoted in the nation's press in his campaign to regulate drug manufacturers and to force price controls on them. Here are just a few examples of Sen. Pryor's tantrum against the industry as reported in various publications:

"The despicable behavior (of the drug industry) can be characterized as nothing short of repulsive."

"The shameful and unrelenting price increases (of drugs) have reached crisis proportions. Over 5 million people over 55 now say they are having to make choices between food and their prescription drugs and between fuel for their home for heat or paying for prescription drugs. If this is the case, what kind of a country have we become?"

"It has been the pressure of Congress and some outraged consumers that has caused some drug companies to hold down prices. Be assured, as soon as the pressure lets up, prices will skyrocket again."

"Millions of older Americans have to go to sleep at night worrying about whether they will be able to afford the medication that controls their high blood pressure or treats

their diabetes. We wonder when this industry will finally develop some compassion for the older Americans who so desperately need the medications they produce."

Rep. Pete Stark, a California Democrat and close ally of Sen. Pryor in the fight to slam price controls on the drug industry, also has been seeking headlines with outlandish statements about the need to lower prescription-drug costs.

In an article in the Aug. 26, 1992, edition of the *Wall Street Journal*, Rep. Stark stretched the truth broadly about the benefits of holding down the costs of prescription drugs. In the article about the need to reduce drug prices so overall health-care costs can be controlled, Rep. Stark was quoted as saying, "If medical-care inflation can be held to 6 percent (a year) from the current 12 percent, the savings will amount to $250 billion a year."

During the past 10 years, the costs of medical care in the U.S. has not seen an increase of 12 percent. The range has been from 7.6 percent to 10.9 percent. That's a tiny error, however, compared to Rep. Stark's claim of a savings of $250 billion a year if the increase could be held to 6 percent. If the cost of health care were to rise by only 6 percent between 1992 and 1993, which apparently is Rep. Stark's goal, the savings compared to a 12 percent increase would be only $49 billion—a far cry from Rep. Stark's $250 billion.

Many consumer-advocate groups also are attacking the industry with ludicrous claims. In a Sept. 10, 1992, report by Families USA Foundation of Washington, D.C., it was stated: "The problem of payment (for prescription drugs by consumers) is expected to worsen in the upcoming years. More and more physicians are electing drug therapy instead of surgery or other costly procedures. However, drugs ***are not cost-effective*** if they are unaffordable."

If drug therapy is less expensive than surgery, and it cures the illness, how is it possible not to be cost-effective?

Under the "Common-Sense Solution," prescription drugs will be both cost-effective and affordable. Consumers would pay for the drugs they can afford and the government-insurance plan would cover the cost of the drugs they can't afford. It would be a disaster to cripple the drug industry with price controls and other regulatory laws in a futile attempt to be compassionate.

The federal government already has tried to impose price controls on prescription drugs sold to Medicaid patients, but the ambitious program backfired almost immediately. A bill, introduced in Congress by Sen. Pryor and Rep. Ron Wyden, an Oregon Democrat, was passed in 1990. It restricts the amount drug companies can charge for medicine used by welfare recipients and other poor people covered by Medicaid. The new law required drug firms to charge Medicaid patients no more for drugs than the lowest amount charged to any other buyer.

Because some customers, such as the Department of Veterans Affairs hospitals and some large health-insurance groups, purchase drugs in huge quantities, they had been receiving volume discounts, often as much as 20 percent lower than the retail price of many prescription drugs. These discounted prices were the ones that had to be charged Medicaid patients under the new law.

Instead of lowering the price to Medicaid patients, most drug companies merely eliminated the discount previously offered to large buyers, meaning that the law resulted in lower prices to no one, but it raised the prices for many others.

Price controls in Canada also have resulted in higher drug prices for U.S. citizens. The Canadian government, in an attempt to control costs of its socialized-medicine plan, placed price controls on prescription drugs sold in that country. The rigid regulations stifled the Canadian pharmaceutical industry and resulted in larger supplies of prescription drugs coming from the U.S.

Since the Canadian restrictions went into effect in 1969, the Canadian drug industry has produced virtually no important new prescription drugs.

U.S. drug companies had no choice but to sell drugs at lower prices to Canadians, and to make up for the difference, U.S. consumers have had to pay higher costs than they would if Canada had a free-market system.

A study by the U.S. General Accounting Office, ordered by Rep. Henry Waxman, a California Democrat, showed that prescription drugs cost an average of 32 percent more in the U.S. than in Canada.

Rep. Waxman pointed out that the study has "once again shown that the U.S. is behind the rest of the world in providing health care to our people. Canada has found ways to control prescription drug prices."

Yes, it's true that the Canadian government has found a way to control drug costs, but these price controls have prevented important progress by Canadian drug manufacturers and has forced cost-shifting to U.S. consumers. Canada isn't the only country with price controls on prescription drugs. The United States is the only Western nation that doesn't have rigid limits on the cost of drugs, and because U.S. manufacturers are major suppliers in all of these nations, there is naturally a great amount of cost-shifting to American consumers.

Shifting of medical costs from one segment of users to another produces no overall benefits. Myron D. Winkelman, a senior vice president at ValueRx Pharmacy Program, Inc., a division of Value Health, Inc., which manages drug-benefit programs for several large corporations, described it succinctly in a Jan. 27, 1992, article in *Business Week* magazine. He said: "It's like squeezing a balloon. Squeeze (prices) at one end, and they pop out somewhere else."

Despite the fact that a system of government-dictated prices fails whenever it is tried, U.S. politicians are determined to pursue their attempts to control drug costs. Twice in the last couple of years, Sen. Pryor has attempted to push his "Prescription Drug Cost Containment Act" through Congress. So far, he has failed, but new attempts are expected.

Sen. Pryor's bill will increase federal income taxes to drug companies if they increase drug prices. Drug firms would see their tax breaks reduced by up to 20 percent for each percentage point that drug prices increase above the inflation rate.

If Congress passes this price-control bill, and if other third-party regulators are successful in reducing prescription drug prices, it could devastate a system that has produced hundreds of important new medicines in past years.

The first casualty will be the expensive research and development efforts that U.S. drug manufacturers are currently engaged in to find cures for cancer, AIDS, heart problems, Alzheimer's and other serious illnesses. It's this unrelenting search for new drugs that has caused most price increases in recent years.

The Pharmaceutical Manufacturers Association claims that drug makers spend an average of $231 million (and more than 10 years) to bring each new drug to market. These costs include developing the drug, testing it for years on animals and then humans, and finally the costly and time-consuming process of getting it approved by the U.S. Food and Drug Administration (FDA).

Currently only two out of every 10 drugs developed by U.S. companies receive FDA approval, and of those that are approved, only three of every 10 are successful enough to recover the original research and development costs.

The amount spent on research and development by all U.S. drug manufacturers has doubled every five years for the past two decades and will exceed more than $11 billion in 1993.

The all-out attack on drug makers in recent years definitely isn't being ignored by the pharmaceutical companies. Most of them are desperately attempting to lower their overhead costs so they can hold down prices of their drugs in an effort to prevent new price-control laws.

Many of the drug manufacturers already have been raising prices less than anticipated or have been lowering prices, adversely affecting profits.

Some of the actions being taken by drug companies were outlined in a Nov. 6, 1992, article in *Business Week*. The magazine pointed out that Bristol-Myers Squibb has announced it will cut 2,300 jobs, or 6 percent of its payroll. Warner-Lambert is planning to trim 2,700 of its 35,000 jobs by 1996. Syntex also is planning layoffs, although no figures have been announced. Merck is planning to shrink its sales staff through attrition. Rhone-Poulenc Rorer has already eliminated 1,000 jobs, and Eli Lilly is planning a restructuring after posting a $269 million third-quarter loss, the company's first loss in more than 30 years.

On Nov. 26, 1992, Monsanto Co. announced it was reducing its total employment by 10 percent, or about 3,200 jobs, with most of the cutbacks occurring at its pharmaceutical subsidiary, G. D. Searle & Co., based in Skokie, Ill. Searle will be losing nearly one-quarter of its work force of 10,000 employees, and it will be making severe reductions in its research and development program.

Monsanto's chief executive officer, Richard Mahoney, said, "Consumers worldwide are demanding products and services at dramatically lower prices. We must respond in this fiercely competitive environment by significantly reducing our cost of doing business."

Viren Mehta of Mehta & Isaly, a New York firm specializing in the study of drug industry operations, told the *New York Times* after the Monsanto announcement: "The whole pharmaceutical industry has come to realize that it had it quite easy in the past, and everyone, even the ones that haven't said so, is busy cost-cutting."

Several companies have pledged to keep drug-price increases at or below the rate of inflation.

The reaction of drug firms to the threat of government price controls and consumer outrage has impacted severely on the stock market, and drug stocks as a group dropped 17 percent in value during the first nine months of 1992. This is highly unusual for an industry that often leads the stock market in gains. Falling stock prices could result in drug companies finding it more difficult to raise capital for expansion.

The drug industry is becoming divided in how to best cope with the problems being forced on it by outsiders. Michael Waldholz, a reporter for the *Wall Street Journal*, described a meeting of industry leaders in a Sept. 25, 1992, article. He wrote: "Early this month, captains of the pharmaceutical industry gathered in Washington, D.C., to grapple with the thorniest problem facing drug companies these days: how to calm rising public ire over the high cost of prescriptions.

"At a special closed meeting of the Pharmaceutical Manufacturers' Association board of directors, chief executives of several companies, including Johnson & Johnson and Glaxo Holdings Ltd., found themselves pitted against those at Merck & Co., Pfizer, Inc., and others. The two factions argued, often vigorously, over how to resist proposed legislation in Congress requiring steep discounts in prices for drugs paid by government health agencies.

" 'The issue caused a split unlike any I've seen in the industry in years,' says a PMA board member who asked not to be identified. 'The specter (of price regulation) has everyone upset.' "

There is little doubt deep trouble lies ahead for the drug industry, and the losers are certain to be U.S. consumers. Here is an industry that has performed amazingly well when left alone to manage its very responsible duties, but when politicians and other outsiders attempt to regulate the companies, trouble erupts from all sides.

Returning the drug industry to the free-market system under the concept of the "Common-Sense Solution" is the only answer.

Index

A

B

C

D

E

F

G

H

N

O

P

R

S

T

U

If you agree that this common-sense solution to the country's medical cost crisis does, indeed, make common sense, you might want to help spread the message.

Quantity discounts are available for bulk purchases of this book.

Please contact:

Bond Publishing Co.
537 East Vine Street
Owatonna, MN 55060

or call toll free:
1-800-374-6888